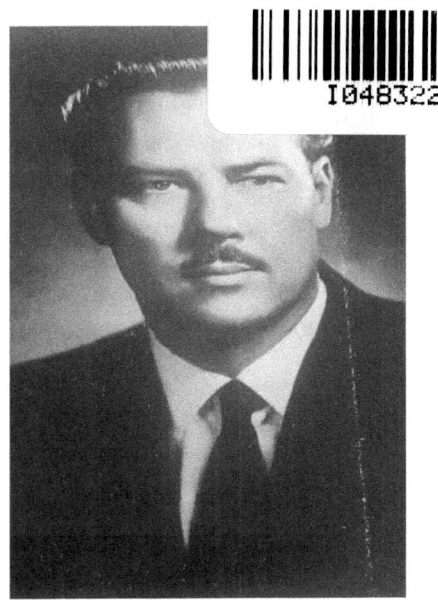

George E. Schauf, M.A., M.D. is the author of the books *Think, Eat and Lose* Fat (Information Inc, 1970), and *Think Thin* (Fawcett 1976). He is the author of *The QQF Theory* for the *Etiology of Obesity*, published in the Journal of American Geriatrics Society in 1973. His paper, *"The Caloric Theory Does Not Apply to Obesity,"* was published in the Journal of the International Academy of Preventive Medicine in 1976, Dr. Schauf is a diplomate of the American Board of Family Practice and a diplomate of the American Board of Bariatric medicine.

In memory of my daughter, Caroline.

...those objects are most profitable to us which can so feed and nourish the body so that all its parts are able to properly preform their functions. For the more capable, the body is of being affected in many ways, the more capable of thinking is the mind...and it is consequently necessary for the requisite nourishment of the body to use many different kinds of food...

—   Baruch Spinoza

George E. Schauf, M.A., M.D.

THE CALORIE CONSPIRACY

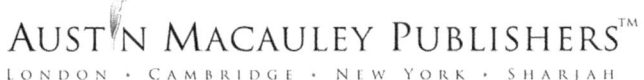

AUSTIN MACAULEY PUBLISHERS™
LONDON • CAMBRIDGE • NEW YORK • SHARJAH

Ordering Information:
Quantity sales: special discounts are available on quantity purchases by corporations, associations, and others. For details, contact the publisher at the address below.

Publisher's Cataloging-in-Publication data
Schauf, M.A., M.D., George E.
The Calorie Conspiracy

ISBN 9781647500252 (Paperback)
ISBN 9781647500269 (Hardback)
ISBN 9781647500276 (ePub e-book)

Library of Congress Control Number: 2020916575

www.austinmacauley.com/us

First Published (2020)
Austin Macauley Publishers LLC
40 Wall Street, 28th Floor
New York, NY 10005
USA

mail-usa@austinmacauley.com
+1 (646) 5125767

20200918

The author wishes to express his deep gratitude to all of those who, in ways, direct or indirect, helped to form his thinking which made this work a reality.

To his teachers and colleagues, for passing on the torch of medical knowledge.

To his patients, from whom many valuable insights were derived.

To this country of ours, for the opportunity to freely express ideas.

To the great American scientists, upon whom the thesis rests.

To the publishers, for their willingness and cooperation in bringing this message to the people.

In particular, he thanks, Marg Dugo, for her maximum efforts in and retyping over and again of the original manuscript.

A special note of thanks to his daughter, Veronica, for her able assistance in the formative stages of the final revisions of this book.

Table of Contents

Introduction

The woman who came into my office in July 1965 was five feet, five inches tall and weighed 232 pounds. At age thirty-four, she measured 50-43-54 and looked to be age forty or older. She carried the misery caused by physical repulsiveness—a deep mental and emotional anguish. For years, she had suffered the tortures of being fat. Her life had been an alienation from social acceptance, and it was in this state of exile that she decided to seek help from a "fat doctor."

I refer to her now because she was typical in some ways of the obese individual seeking assistance and because her visit occurred at about the time, I decided to write this book.

Many of my patients have been very fat. The treatment that restored her to health and attractiveness will not only work for people who are only slightly fatter than they should be, but it works for extreme cases such as my typical patients.

Notice that I use the term "fat," not "overweight." "Overweight" is a misconception. More about that later.

In the interest of identification, I shall call this woman Jane.

In over fifty years of family practice, the last forty of which have been devoted in large part to the treatment of obesity and related problems, I have seen literally hundreds of Janes and their male counterparts come through my door. Many of these people had failed at various diet-control and/or weight-reducing programs related to, or stemming from the caloric theory—the theory adhered to by most physicians. Many of these patients, frustrated and disillusioned, had heard that I was successfully treating obesity with a different set of rules.

What I told Jane—what I tell every patient during the initial visit—was that I did not follow the popularly accepted treatment for obesity: the restriction of calories. That approach is very general and nonspecific and has been proven ineffectual. The amount of food we consume is only part of the story. The kind of foods and the frequency of meals are equally important.

The term "weight," in any case, is ambiguous. For example, if you entered a hardware or grocery store and asked the clerk for "eight pounds," I'm sure the person behind the counter would reply, "Eight pounds of what?"

Many physicians today are telling their patients to lose ten, twenty, or thirty pounds, but not saying what the pounds to be lost are made of. Are they pounds of fat, of water, or of essential lean tissues?

My treatment, I told Jane, is designed to rid the body of excess fat, and simultaneously to rebuild the lean body tissues such as muscles, liver, kidney, glands, blood, and other vital body parts. Thus, the general body efficiency will be increased.

Severe caloric restriction results in a loss of muscles and other vital tissues, which shows up as sunken face and sagging tissue, for instance. Several of my patients, following my system, have lost as much as eighty pounds in one year—twelve to thirteen inches in bust, waist, and hip measurements—*by eating more instead of less*, ultimately appearing years younger and feeling enormously improved.

In recent years, there have been several significant findings regarding obesity from medical research. After exhaustive studies, my program of treatment has been initiated. Here, I will attempt to explain only the elementary principles.

In general, your brain must have blood sugar (glucose) at all times. The body can turn lean tissue proteins into glucose but cannot, repeat cannot turn your body fat into glucose. In the past, some physicians, creditable men, influenced by the caloric theory, have sincerely but erroneously informed their patients that *they can stop eating and "live on" their fat surplus.* Unfortunately, the brain cannot utilize the surplus fat. Consequently, if you do not eat, the body, responding to the glucose needs of the brain, will arbitrarily mutate your muscle, liver, kidney, or something equally vital into glucose. By starving, you will develop progressively weaker and thinner muscles and may develop anemia and other maladies due to the loss of vital tissues.

The primary source of energy to the muscles of your body is fat, in the form of free fatty acid. *Therefore, to lose this fat, exercise becomes vitally important.* Many overweight people, however, cannot exercise productively because of a weakened muscular condition, or extreme fat accumulation, and therefore certain medications may be necessary. Such cases should be under the close care of a doctor.

People should remember that the scale is only one measurement. In actuality, the best way to judge physical harmony is by your mirror reflection and by the way you feel. The use of the tape measure *is actually a much more accurate measure of body fat loss than is the scale.*

The diet you will be on, my explanation to Jane continued, will restrict the daily carbohydrates to between 45 and 70 grams a day. "You must eat three meals and two between-meal snacks per day. And, do not leave the table feeling hungry. You must have some protein at each meal, chosen from the animal products: eggs, meat, fish, chicken, and cheese.

"You must eat more omega-3 essential fats since every cell in the body contains necessary fat molecules, and free fatty acids are the major source of aerobic energy to the muscles and other vital lean tissues, including the heart. The fat you eat does not of itself turn into body fat since it is impossible to store body fat without the presence of alpha-glycerophosphate, which is a glucose metabolite, and insulin, which is secreted by the body in response to a rise in blood sugar above the normal. You will be given a physical examination and blood tests will be drawn from which several basic lab screening tests can be measured. These include tests for blood sugar, serum cholesterol, serum triglycerides, kidney function, liver function, thyroid function, and a complete blood count. You may require certain medications according to my clinical evaluation and the results of your lab tests."

I concluded with Jane by wishing her success during the treatment program, by encouraging her to carry out the dietary plan even though it may be contrary to what she had always heard and believed. Of course, she harbored doubts, and justifiably so. It simply didn't make sense to her. She is five feet five, weighs 232, feels ugly and rejected, and I have just suggested that she eat more, not less! Like many, she is dubious about entering the program.

I think, basically, that Jane's uncertainty, which ultimately proved to be wrong, and the happiness and improved state of health reached by Jane and other patients, are what motivated me to write this book. And, it had to do with the misery suffered by the obese and the deep shadows in which they circulate, seeking help.

Jane decided to try the program. The progress, which we shall examine later on, was astonishing.

People use the term "weight" as the word for what they want to lose.

But what is "weight?"

The human body consists of three essential components: (1) water, (2) body fat, and (3) lean body tissues in muscles, glands, liver, kidney, and so on. We are capable of losing or gaining weight in any one of these components—and the scale will register the pounds lost or acquired, but cannot tell us whether it was body fat, extracellular fluids, or essential lean body tissue.

During the past several decades, there have been dramatic and revolutionary advances in the field of metabolic research. I have microscopically examined medical literature during my engagement with obesity work and have, coupling this information with my own patients' results, evolved a new theory for the cause of obesity and formulated a successful method for *losing fat and keeping it off permanently.*

If you are trying to lose "weight," this book has the answer to your problem.

Chapter I

A New Theory Regarding Obesity

If you have a "weight" problem, this will interest you. It is a departure from calorie counting as a way of losing body fat.

The caloric theory—if the number of calories we consume exceeds the number of calories expended as the energy, we will gain weight, and if vice versa, we lose weight—has been the accepted "truth" for the cause and treatment of obesity for several decades.

It's not really known who originated this theory, but it came into acceptance in the very beginning of metabolic research, when the crude bomb calorimeter had been invented and researchers were able, for the first time, to determine that in each gram of fat, there were nine calories, in each gram of protein four calories, and in each gram of carbohydrate, four calories.

There is no question that *the caloric theory is a gross oversimplification and actually a distortion of the facts* concerning a problem that is vexing the lives of over ninety million Americans today. In view of new medical-research findings plus long-established knowledge, it is now apparent that the caloric theory has become obsolete.

A calorie is a measurement of heat energy. Kerosene, diesel, and gasoline all liberate calories, but hardly can be utilized interchangeably as fuels. *Protein, fat, and carbohydrate all liberate calories but are by no means used interchangeably by the body.*

Cotton, lead, and rubber all have weight, but it is necessary to differentiate among them. Since the body has three essential components—vital lean tissues in muscle, water, and body fat—it is equally necessary to determine in which component we lose or gain weight. The bathroom scale cannot tell us that. Most people, preoccupied with scale weight, understandably may assume any lost weight has been body fat. This is not always the case, as is clearly demonstrated in cases of starvation, where wasted muscle tissue is shown in an emaciated facial expression, sagging skin from thin limbs, and a sunken chest.

Doctors Michael Ball and Lawrence Kyle of the Georgetown University School of Medicine at Washington, D.C., conducted exhaustive studies that have demonstrated unequivocally that weight loss can be vital tissue, water, or body fat according to changing conditions of diet and exercise.

In a crude way, the caloric theory has suggested that the human body is a burning barrel; whatever goes into the barrel must be burned or its weight increases.

I prefer comparing the human body to an automobile since this comparison will lend nicely toward an understanding of how the body uses food as energy. In the auto, there are *two primary sources* of energy: gasoline and electricity. The "gasoline" of your body is fat in the form of free fatty acid, and your "electricity" is carbohydrate in the form of blood sugar (glucose). Your "battery" is the liver and your "gas tank" your body fat, and the muscles your "hybrid engine" (Figure A).

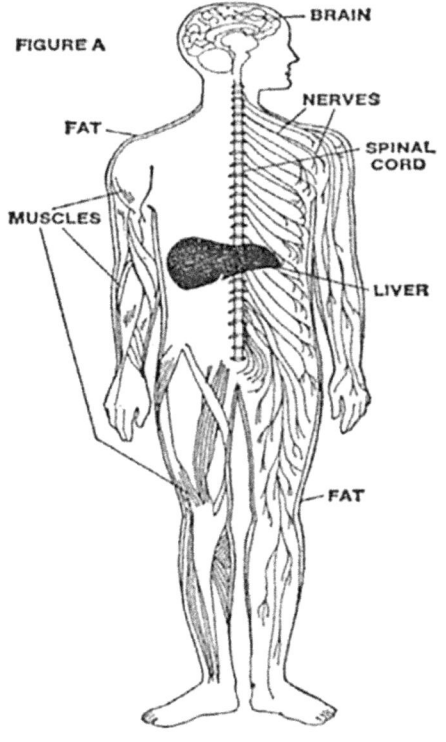

FIGURE A

This figure illustrates the dual-energy system of the human body. Glucose stored in the liver is the mandatory energy of the brain and nerves. Body fat stored beneath the skin is the primary aerobic energy to the muscles and other lean tissues. Glucose stored as glycogen in the muscles is alternative energy to the muscles during oxygen debt.

You may have heard people say that they had to have their batteries recharged. What they really meant was that they had to have the liver's glycogen supply replenished with sugar (glucose). The total storage capacity of the liver glycogen rarely exceeds 200-300 calories, enough to keep the "light," your brain, and the "ignition system," your nerves, functioning for three to four hours. The obligatory source of energy to your brain and nervous system is blood sugar (glucose). Because the liver's capacity to store glucose as glycogen is limited, this supply must be maintained at all times.

The great majority of your other tissues—muscles, kidneys, heart, and other organs—use fat in the form of free fatty acid as their primary aerobic energy source. This is an excellent form of energy since it is stored as nine calories per gram and is an almost unlimited quantity. It is readily available to the muscles requiring great amounts of energy. The fat that you eat is stored, then liberated from the fat cells in the form of free fatty acid, the aerobic energy to the muscles. *Measurement of the exact amount of fat oxidized as energy has been a difficult technical task.*

Just as the lights, radio, and ignition of an auto consume electricity stored in the battery, your brain and nerves consume glucose stored in your battery, the liver. The power source of an auto, the engine, burns gasoline stored in the gas tank. The power source of your body, the muscles, burn fat scored under the skin and adjacent to the muscle using it. The muscles will burn sugar (glucose) that is stored as muscle glycogen in states of prolonged exercise where available oxygen is insufficient to meet energy demands.

To understand more clearly the significance of this hybrid "duo" energy system, visualize a car with a 100-gallon gasoline tank mounted on its roof. Obviously, this extra weight would cause undue strain on the tires, shock absorbers, and bearings, and would hinder the car from accelerating. Now, suppose that each day, a wire or sparkplug was removed from the engine. In a short while, this car would lose all of its go-power. People who carry a "100-gallon gasoline tank" around in the form of excess body fat and are daily losing vital parts by starving themselves (vital tissues are mutilated during starvation to supply the necessary glucose to the brain) and likewise lose their go-power.

However, it must be emphasized that *the food you eat not only supplies energy,* but *the great bulk of it is used to maintain and repair the body cells* that make up your vital structural parts—tissues and organs such as muscles, blood, kidneys, glands, and so on. These vital body parts are composed mainly of protein units called amino acids. *At least 60 to 70 grams of protein in the diet per day are needed just to maintain and repair body tissue.* Aside from protein, your body also requires fat units, called fatty acids, as structural and integral parts of the cell membrane of all vital body cells. Every cell of your body, including your vital body hormones, contains cholesterol and a fat protein complex called lipoprotein as an integral part of the cell structure.

Another experiment conducted at the Oakland Naval Hospital and described in the *Annals of Internal Medicine* in October 1965 has proven dramatically that starvation will result in weight loss, but largely at the expense of vital tissues. *Obese seamen* who had been starved ten days lost twenty pounds, but it was shown that 65 percent, or *thirteen pounds,* of the weight that they had lost while starving was vital lean tissue. The same seamen on a very low carbohydrate diet lost less weight but twice the amount of body fat and only .4 of a pound of lean tissue.

The proven experiences of most people who have reduced by the method of severely restricting calories have lost "weight," but in almost all instances regain the "weight" they have lost, and then some. And they regain it as unwanted fat.

Since all dietary carbohydrates become blood sugar, necessary to our brain and nerves, why must we limit carbohydrates in our diet? You realize that excessive carbohydrate intake causes the blood sugar to rise to levels that induce the secretion of insulin from the pancreas. *Insulin will cause blood sugar* to be changed to fat at the cell membrane of every fat cell in the body, of which there are countless millions. Proteins are largely utilized as cellular structures but if eaten in excess can also be converted to glucose and promote insulin secretion by the pancreas with subsequent storage of body fat. Therefore, free access to meat and fish is to be avoided. Moderation is the key, promoted by limiting the proteins to 3-5 ounces per meal

The frequency of your meals is also important. The continued process of adding fat to your body and tearing down vital tissue by eating one large meal a day will cause you to develop sarcopenic obesity and become a "skinny" person inside a heavy coat of fat. As the load increases and your body muscles and other vital tissues become depleted, your activity will correspondingly be decreased. You may be continually tired and find you have less and less energy to engage in physical exercise, which promotes the burning and loss of body fat. In fact, *physical exercise is the best way to rid yourself of excess body fat.* It increases the rate at which your muscles and other body cells burn fat as energy. But in order to exercise so as to lose fat, your muscles should be performing at peak efficiency. *Since starving or eating only one large meal per day causes you to lose muscle mass, you may not be able to exercise enough to cause significant fat loss.*

For any reducing diet, you should consider three integral factors—the quality of food you eat, the quantity of food you eat, and the frequency of your meals.

The kind of quality of the food you eat is important since your primary aim is to nourish your body, the hormones, enzymes, and cells, etc., of the vital lean tissues (largely composed of protein amino acid and essential omega-3 and omega 6-fats) and to stop storing more body fat. The amount of food you eat—particularly of the carbohydrates—is important for if excessive will add to your outer coat of fat. The *frequency of meals* is important to prevent excess fat storage, the loss of muscle and other vital lean tissues, and therefore to prevent sarcopenic obesity.

I have published the aforementioned concepts under the formula QQF: quality, quantity, and frequency—the new theory concerning the cause of obesity. It was published and presented in a number of medical journals and at a number of national medical conventions which are listed in the appendix.

I shall elaborate upon the QQF theory later on. At this point, let me suggest that you "think thin" and "eat to live, not live to eat."

The method of dieting to be illustrated in subsequent chapters is designed to rid your body of excess body fat while rebuilding and maintaining your vital lean tissues. Once your excessive body fat has been lost, it will not be regained if you will remain on the way of eating outlined in this book. By feeding your vital lean tissues while starving the fat cells, you will become that trim, healthy, and attractive person you've always wanted to be.

Chapter II
The Obesity Problem

For a number of years, it was assumed that obesity was simply a matter of overeating and that the solution to the problem was simply to reduce the number of calories in the diet. The clinical experience of many physicians has taught them otherwise. Though observing patients who overate without becoming fat and others who held themselves on near-starvation diets without losing weight, it became apparent that there must be something more to this problem and that a true explanation of obesity was to be obtained by a basic understanding of the underlying metabolic mechanisms of the body. Some of these were described in the previous chapter.

Many obese patients who feel compelled to eat are not undisciplined, emotionally unbalanced gluttons suffering from a lack of gratification, as many have been accused of being, but rather are actually hungry and are eating to satisfy the very real need for essential fats and proteins. Many times, the method of treatment being urged upon them— cutting down calories and restriction of high-calorie dietary fats—*has added to their problem*, for it has promoted the loss of vital lean tissues more than it has caused them to lose body fat. Indeed, *it has been a self-defeating system*. The lean tissues burn fat as energy. Thus, when losing lean tissue, the body has a lessened capacity to "burn" its accumulated fat.

Obesity is a multi-faceted problem, really, involving the total person. Obviously, *it is caused by improper eating habits* probably stemming from ignorance of what constitutes a well-balanced diet. Compulsive eating, particularly of carbohydrates, is a sure-fire cause. Other factors involved are the personality of the individual, his psychological needs, his heredity, his general health, the status of the endocrine or glandular system; the abundance, variety, and attractiveness of available foods (here again, particularly the sugars and starches); advertising of food via the communications media, environmental stress, internal conflicts, and the amount of physical exercise he or she indulges in. Since there are also other factors involved in obesity, it becomes obvious that it is highly complex and that the simple treatment of counting calories to overcome it, is markedly oversimplified and has become obsolete.

Types of Obesity

Let us consider, for a moment, the categories of obese people. Generally, there are two. The first, *the over-nourished obese,* includes those people who are compulsive overeaters. Probably, they have failed at several attempts to reduce, may have tried various diets or read a book or two on the subject, but they continue to eat all foods in excess. These people may have healthy bodies but have accumulated excess body fat.

The second category, the *undernourished obese*, are those people who have been chronically exposed to an unbalanced diet. Under various environmental pressures, they usually decide to diet by limiting the high-calorie, fat and protein-plus-fat foods, choosing to subsist on the low-calorie foods, which are largely starches and sugars. Though "overweight," they are actually in a state of malnutrition, having excessive body fat, but with depleted vital tissues—muscles, kidneys, liver, and so on.

A distinction between these two general categories is made because many times, the advice to lose "weight" by reducing caloric intake is heeded by the obese person, yet he finds that although he tries to reduce his caloric intake—and he may be successful—he just cannot succeed in losing weight, and at times may even gain! This condition may be a reflection upon a glandular system in an unbalanced state, but it most often indicates a condition of vital-lean-tissue depletion and fluid retention.

Many may register initial weight loss by the method of caloric restriction, but almost *invariably will regain* what they have lost, and then some.

Counting calories is a yo-yo up-and-down affair. The loss of weight may be only temporary and quickly regained.

Stages of Obesity

Aside from the two general categories, there are different stages of obesity within any one person. These stages depend upon the total internal environment of the body, particularly the status of the endocrine glandular system, chronological age, sex, duration of improper eating habits, amount of physical exercise, and the various environmental stresses one may be subjected to. A final stage, the so-called resistant obese, are those who hold their weight no matter how much they cut down calories.

It has been experimentally shown that obese persons have nearly three times as many fat cells as do lean people. In the stages of obesity from infancy to adulthood, new fat cells are produced. Since every fat cell is a miniature fat factory, it becomes increasingly easier to produce and store fat as the condition of obesity progresses. *The fatter you are the easier it is to get fatter.* However, if you are fat there is no need to despair. The way of eating presented in this book is designed in particular to help those people who are already fat, but it will also prevent countless thousands from becoming obese.

Types of Body Fat

Clinical examination of obese patients has revealed several distinct types of body-fat distribution. *One frequent type* occurs in what could be described as the active-dynamic kind of person, the majority of whom seem to be women. She is well-liked, pleasant, and apparently very energetic. Usually, her body tissue is firm, with a prominence of *fat distribution on the thigh* about ten inches below the hip joint. Some physicians have classified this type of person as one in whom the *pituitary gland* is secreting relatively over-actively, and who demonstrates periodic low blood sugar due to the over-secretion of insulin. (This pattern of fat distribution has been noted in juvenile diabetics who chronically receive insulin.) If this condition goes unrecognized and untreated, after many years this person's firm, resilient tissue will degenerate and become flabby and redundant, a condition resulting from relative under-activity of the pituitary gland due to its exhaustion.

Another type of fat distribution, the hypogonadal, appears as a marked fat accumulation occurring on the hips above the hip joint, on the abdomen and buttocks. There may be a decrease in breast size in women, which often occurs in women suffering an ovarian deficiency due to surgical extirpation of the ovaries or to postmenopausal conditions. Male hypogonadal types have excess fat on the buttocks and in the breast area.

The person who measures approximately the same at chest, abdomen, and hips may have a relative thyroid deficiency.

People who develop a *fat pad over the posterior shoulder area* are commonly referred to as having a *"buffalo hump."* This particular fat distribution is associated with over-activity of the adrenal glands and occurs in patients who have been on prolonged treatment with cortisone. Other characteristics of this type are increased weight in the abdomen, upper arms, and chest. The face may be ruddy with "chipmunk" jowls. Purplish lines will mark their abdomens.

Lastly, a body-weight distribution commonly seen is that in the person whose body appears *slender and normal from the waist up, while the bulk of his weight is in the lower extremities.* These people usually are conscious of their legs and tend to draw less attention to them by inactivity. This only aggravates the condition, since it tends toward water accumulation and increased swelling.

When a *specific type of body-fat distribution* appears in the obese patient, chances are that it *is related in some way to an imbalance of the biochemical and glandular functions.* People with such problems should seek the care of a specialist.

In those who chronically indulge in carbohydrates, there may be no definite fat distribution, but they are always generously laden with body fat.

Advances in Treatment

The current treatment of obesity which has been used by the majority of physicians in the past is caloric restriction, usually in conjunction with an appetite suppressant and a diuretic—the idea being that all calories must be metabolized and therefore, if we eat fewer calories than we metabolize, we will lose "weight." In view of recent advances in the study of carbohydrate and fat metabolism, this theory strikes me as a gross oversimplification. My own methods and rationale were arrived at from these recent research findings. A more meaningful way *to think of food* is to consider the *three different types—proteins, fat, and carbohydrate*—and to consider the different manner in which the body utilizes them.

Many times, the system of calorie counting may actually promote an excess caloric intake since the calorie-counting method is a form of mental conditioning that creates a preoccupation with the desire for food, which will often lead to rebellion and subsequent overeating.

In fact, however popularly accepted the caloric restriction program has been, the great majority of obese people who have tried this system have failed.

Telling a person to push himself away from the table or limit himself to 1,000 calories daily has been an ineffective method; the concentration has been too severely centered upon the quantity of food ingested, almost disregarding the quality and frequency of meals.

Let's remember that the causes of obesity are many, the most prominent being improper eating habits and lack of exercise. Most people who have been dieting by the caloric-restriction method have become disillusioned with the results. They exhibit the "yo-yo syndrome," losing weight by cutting calories only to regain it again when returning to random eating habits.

To Sum Up

1. There are two general categories of obese people: those who continue to eat all foods excessively, and those who attempt to diet by reducing calories subsisting on an unbalanced diet. The latter, though obese, are actually suffering from malnutrition and usually demonstrate a low metabolism with excessive body fat but depleted lean tissues in muscle, liver, etc., This group, according to my clinical experience, comprises the majority of overweight people. Those with excessive body fat with simultaneous extreme depletion of the lean tissues of muscles, liver, and kidney, etc., have been classified as having sarcopenic obesity.

2. Certain distinct fat distributions in obese people are related to glandular and biochemical imbalances. They should be treated by an endocrinologist.

Chapter III

Your Food

To arrive at any logical basis for dieting, knowledge of what you are eating is essential. Generally, food is composed of proteins, fats, carbohydrates, vitamins, minerals, water, and fiber. A better understanding of food is key to overcoming obesity.

Proteins

These are derived chiefly from animal sources: meat, fish, fowl, eggs, cheese, and milk. We call the animal proteins complete, or good proteins because they contain all the vital amino acids our bodies cannot manufacture. Similarly, complete *vegetable proteins* are found in *soybeans, yeast, wheat germ, and corn germ.* There are also many sources of "incomplete" proteins, which either lack or are relatively deficient in some of the essential amino acids. Incomplete animal-sourced proteins are found in egg whites and in gelatin. Incomplete vegetable proteins are present in lima beans, navy beans, peas, cereals, wheat gluten, and flour. I make the distinction between complete and incomplete proteins because all of the essential amino acids must be present at one time in a package before they can be manufactured into body tissue. Incomplete proteins can be converted to blood sugar to sustain the brain and nervous system between meals, but of themselves, they are less valuable as tissue builders than are animal proteins. When taken in the proper combinations, however, they do become valuable tissue builders.

Table I

Minimal requirements of the eight essential amino acids

Grams per day

Amino Acids	Minimal Requirements
Tryptophan	25
Phenylalanine	1.10
Lysine	0.80
Threonine	0.50
Valine	0.80
Methionine	1.10
Isoleucine	0.70
Leucine	1.10

Biochemical units from which protein molecules are formed are called amino acids. The amino acids are the building blocks of the body structure. Of the twenty-three different amino acids, eight are essential and must be taken in the diet, since the body cannot manufacture them. (See Table I.) Though the variety of order and frequency of their appearance, and the nature of the chemical links between them, the twenty-three amino acids form an almost *limitless* number of protein compounds. *The entire body structure "is" protein*; when we stop to think of the hair, skin, muscles, eyes, brain, lungs, stomach, intestines, and other organs all being composed of different arrangements of amino acids, it is a marvel indeed. Aside from body structure, the enzymes of the internal body machinery that permit the oxidation of energy sources vital to the life process itself are proteins. The hormones are lipoproteins. The blood carries on its vital function through protein. The antibodies that protect the body against infection are protein. Even the enzymes that digest our food are protein. In fact, the uses of the body for protein are protean, to coin a pun.

Is it any wonder, then, that if you avoid protein, your body efficiency will be greatly decreased?

Protein also serves as a major source of energy as it is converted to sugar in the liver. This conversion may be from the protein you take at mealtime or, if not available in your diet, from your body tissue itself, since protein, except as functioning body parts, is not stored. Because of growth and the aging process, the cells of the body are in a perpetual state of change, and proteins, therefore, must be ingested in adequate daily amounts to meet the various body needs. *At least sixty to seventy grams of protein must be eaten per day just to maintain and repair body tissues.*

The two main proteins in the *blood plasma are albumin and globulin.*

Albumin acts to regulate the blood volume and further is an important carrier in the transport of various substances.

With particular reference to obesity, *albumin* is the necessary carrier for free fatty acids as they are transferred in the bloodstream to the muscles and other vital tissues, where they are used as aerobic energy. The globulin proteins form antibodies that act to defend against various infective agents.

These plasma proteins, albumin, and globulin, are in a constant state of dynamic equilibrium with the surrounding tissue. That is, the tissue proteins and plasma proteins are being continually interchanged according to whatever conditions are in effect at a given time. This explains how blood-serum measurements of proteins can be within the normal range in a person while his body tissue proteins may be generally depleted.

One clinical condition that seems to result from general protein-tissue depletion is edema, or accumulation of water in the tissues, which often appears in obese people who have severely limited their caloric intake. Their *tissues are water-logged.* This water may be intracellular or extracellular, depending upon the other factors that affect the blood level of various hormones and electrolytes. Other conditions resulting from general protein-tissue depletion are decreased mobility of the bowels (due to swelling of the bowel lining with water), with subsequent constipation; increased susceptibility to infection, anemia, and delayed wound healing. *In alcoholics who do not eat, protein deficiency in their diet will result in the loss of vital liver cells and lead to cirrhosis of the liver.*

From having treated and observed many obese patients, I have concluded that countless complaints of fatigue, backache, indigestion, and myalgia stem from protein-depleted tissues.

Why are proteins important in treating obesity? As we have seen in starvation or extreme caloric restriction, over 50% of weight loss is essential vital tissue. Since vital tissues burn fat as their major energy source, these tissues must be maintained at their full capacity in order to burn and lose the maximum amount of body fat. Also, eating sufficient protein is the way to assure ample glucose energy to the brain and nerves between meals. If not in excess, proteins can be converted to sugar (glucose) in the liver without causing a blood-sugar rise and subsequent fat production. The resulting pep necessary to engage in physical exercise, work, and play, will cause fat to be burned as aerobic energy for the muscles and other vital lean tissues. In order to become healthy and trim a *daily and adequate, but not excessive, ingestion of protein is mandatory.*

Fats

This frightening little word is repugnant to the obese person. In medical terminology, fats are called lipids. *Lipids* are organic substances occurring in plants and animals, which are not soluble in water but only in inorganic solvents, such as ether. Lipids include neutral or true fat, phospholipids, lecithins, cephalins, cerebrosides and sterols, the latter including cholesterol. So the word "fat" is actually general and nonspecific and covers a multitude of nutritional substances, many of which serve as vital structural components in the body machinery.

There are two classes of fat; saturated and unsaturated. The proportions of saturated and unsaturated fats as they appear in animal and vegetable sources are listed in Table II on page 37.

The subject of fat has received wide attention over the past several years because of the stated relationship between saturated-fat ingestion and elevated serum cholesterol levels. It has been shown that the ingestion of polyunsaturated fats tends to lower the serum cholesterol, and therefore, it has been theorized, the latter should be eaten almost exclusively to decrease the incidence of heart attacks. *Current medical opinion is not in agreement regarding this supposition, but rather suggests the ingestion of both saturated and unsaturated fat, in a ratio of roughly two unsaturated to one saturated.* Recent clinical evidence indicates that when high amounts of polyunsaturated fats are taken in the diet, Vitamin-E supplements should be taken concurrently.

Ingested fats serve two purposes: to supply energy, and to maintain and build body structure. Most people view *fat as that which bulges in the wrong places, not realizing that fat molecules, particularly the phospholipids, are found in practically all body tissue, especially the muscles.* Certain body enzymes require lipids for their action, and the molecular nucleus that forms many of the essential body hormones is derived from cholesterol. There are certain essential fatty acids our body cannot manufacture, i.e., linolenic acid and linoleic acid so it is vital that our daily diet includes them for good health.

Table II

	Animal Products	Percent Saturated	Percent Unsaturated
Meat	Beef	48	47
	Lamb	56	40
	Luncheon meats	36	59
	Pork	38	58
	Bacon	32	63
	Liver (pork)	34	61
Milk	Cow's milk	55	39
	Goat's milk	62	33
Poultry	Chicken	32	64
	Eggs	32	61
Fish	Herring	19	77
	Salmon	15	79
	Tuna	25	70
Fats & Oils	Butter	55	39
	Lard	38	57
	Codfish liver	17	81
	Halibut liver	17	72
Cereals & Grains	Cornmeal	11	82
	Oats	22	74
	Rice	17	81
	Sorghum	12	81
	Wheat flour (white)	14	76
	Wheat germ	15	77

	Animal Products	Percent Saturated	Percent Unsaturated
Fruits & Vegetables	Avocado pulp	20	69
	Olives	56	39
	Soybeans	20	79
Nuts	Almonds	8	87
	Brazil nuts	20	76
	Cashews	17	17
	Coconut	86	8
	Peanut butter	26	70
	Pecans	7	84
	Walnuts (English)	7	89
Other Fats & Oils	Corn oil	10	84
	Cottonseed oil	25	71
	Margarine	26	70
	Olive oil	11	84
	Peanut oil	18	76
	Safflower oil	8	87
	Shortening (animal)	43	53
	Shortening (vegetable)	23	72
	Soybean oil	12	83

The percentages indicate the relative amount of saturated as compared to unsaturated fat. The actual amount of fat will vary with the particular food.

As stated, the main source of aerobic energy to the body is free fatty acid, available from ingested and/or stored body fat. If you recall the analogy of an automobile, ingested fat, particularly the polyunsaturated kind, acts to prime the body engine and get it going so that the body will burn its stored fat. A mechanic can tell you that when the engine carburetor is dry, pouring a little gasoline into the carburetor will prime it so that the engine will begin burning the fuel from the gas tank. So it is with the body. Vegetable oils act as a primer to get our muscles going, burning more of our unwanted excess body fat. Fat is used as aerobic energy by the muscles (they consume by far the largest percentage of body energy), and by most other body cells. The striking exceptions to this are the brain and nervous system, which cannot use free fatty acid, but instead must use blood sugar (glucose).

Although *fat is a very necessary part of anyone's diet,* it is a common belief that if we eat fat, we will get fat. This is not always true. Experiments have shown that high-fat, low-carbohydrate diets cause twice the amount of body-fat loss as very-low-calorie diets. However, emphasis on the linkage of elevated blood-cholesterol levels with arteriosclerosis has served to scare too many Americans away from eating fat.

It has never been established that cholesterol causes arteriosclerosis; the guilt has been assumed by association. Recent studies have implied that hyperglycemia and hyperinsulinism may be related causal agents and that low-functioning thyroid glands may also play a role in the development of arteriosclerosis. On the other hand, it is an established fact that high concentrations of sugar injected into an artery is damaging to the internal lining of the arteries.

A 1965 experiment at U.C.L.A. isolated a heart cell from an animal heart. Researchers extracted an oily substance from the cell. When this fatty substance was removed, the heart cell stopped beating. Upon replacing the fatty substance, the cell began functioning again. If the human heart behaves likewise, it can be safely deduced that our lives are virtually dependent upon fat.

Carbohydrates

Here are the refined sugars in "sweets"—pies, cookies, candy, cake, soft drinks; natural sugars in fruits; the starches in grains—breads and cereals, and macaroni, etc.; and the vegetable starches in potatoes, lima beans, corn, and peas. A general, but handy, identification tag is this: if the food on your plate didn't come from an animal and if it isn't fat, then it's carbohydrate or contains a goodly percentage of carbohydrate. (A comprehensive list of the gram content of carbohydrates in various foods can be found in the Never After Breakfast Carbohydrate Counter in the appendix.)

When carbohydrates are ingested, they are then digested and assimilated as blood sugar. In contrast to the body's almost limitless storage space for fat—the entire skin envelope—the body's capacity to store sugar in the liver is rarely more than 50-75 grams or 200-300 calories. When this capacity is exceeded, as it frequently is, blood-sugar levels rise and insulin is secreted, transforming blood sugar to body fat almost instantly at the cell membrane of every fat cell in the system. This awesome capacity of the human body to convert blood sugar into fat by the action of insulin at the countless millions of fat cells has been known only during the past four decades. Previously, it was held that the conversion of sugar to fat could occur only in the liver.

It is a paradox that the *brain and nervous system must have blood sugar constantly, although the total storage capacity of sugar in the liver is only 200-300 calories.* Eating carbohydrates is not the way to keep energy *flowing to the brain since excess carbohydrates are continually changed into body fat. But the body has the ability to convert protein into sugar without causing sudden rises that would provoke insulin and fat production.* This will ensure a continued steady source of energy to the brain and nervous system between meals and during complete abstinence from food. Hence, eating protein at each meal is a very effective method for avoiding the between-meal craving for sweets.

In the past, some doctors claimed that we did not require carbohydrates at all. I wouldn't go this far. *If the liver becomes depleted of glycogen (sugar),* it begins making ketone bodies from fat. Ketone bodies are a limited "reserve" energy source to the brain and the nerves. However, if this continues, excess ketone compounds accumulate, which may cause ill health and can induce coma or even death in patients with severe diabetes. We estimate that *daily consumption of about thirty grams of carbohydrates is sufficient* to prevent this condition of excess ketone-body accumulation.

Vitamins

This is a remarkable group of compounds present in minute quantities in a wide range of foods, and necessary for the maintenance of normal health and body growth. They are not *synthesized by the body* and hence *must come from the diet.* Usually, if you eat a well-balanced diet *with variety,* the necessary daily vitamin requirement will be provided. However, because of food processing and improper eating habits, many people today develop deficiencies in vitamins. In cases where it is known that dietary intake is inadequate, vitamin supplements are recommended. This is a normal procedure for obese people who have been restricting their caloric intake over a period of several months.

Vitamins fall into two general classifications: those soluble in water and those soluble in fat. Water-soluble vitamins are not stored by the body to any degree, and therefore their daily intake is mandatory for good health. The fat-soluble vitamins, stored in the liver, require bile salts and fat in order to be absorbed. Consequently, people who drastically limit their intake of fat or have gall-bladder disease may find themselves deficient in fat-soluble.

Vitamin B Complex and C are water-soluble, whereas A, D, E, and K are fat-soluble.

Vitamin A occurs in cod-liver and fish oils, butter, eggs, and cheese. Vegetable sources of carotenes (converted to vitamin A in the body) are carrots, sweet potatoes, squash, pumpkin, apricots, peaches, and yellow corn. Vitamin A is necessary for growth and the maintenance of bones and teeth. The absence of this vitamin will cause drying of the tear ducts, thickening of the lining of the eye socket, scariness, dryness of the skin and night blindness. On the other hand, excess amounts of vitamin A may cause hyperirritability, tender swelling of the bones, itching, and sparse, coarse hair.

The B vitamins include about ten different compounds referred to as B Complex. They are thiamine (vitamin B_1), riboflavin, nicotinic acid (niacin), and pyridoxine (B_6), pantothenic acid, folic acid, inositol, and biotin. Vitamin B Complex is found in yeast, liver, and grain cereals.

Thiamine (B_1) is in good supply in whole grains, legumes, beef, pork, liver, nuts, yeast, and leafy vegetables. It is important mainly in the enzyme processes of carbohydrate metabolism. A deficiency may cause neuritis with varying symptoms, depending upon the extent of the shortage. Some of the early symptoms are mental depression, irritability, poor memory, and tiredness. Later indications are pain in the legs and loss of ability to feel vibrations. This may lead to actual paralysis in extreme cases of thiamine deficiency. Also, in certain extreme situations, a disease called beriberi will occur with the triad of neuritis, enlargement of the heart, and edema, with a swelling of the legs with water caused by heart failure.

Riboflavin is found in milk, meat (especially liver and kidney), fish, eggs, and leafy vegetables. This vitamin is an integral part of the enzyme system in amino-acid metabolism. Deficiencies result in cracking at the corner of the mouth, a red tongue, inflammation of the eyeball socket, a scaly, greasy dermatitis of the face, ears and other areas of the body.

Nicotinic acid (niacin) occurs in liver, fish, milk, eggs, cheese, lean meat, wheat, unpolished rice, and peanuts. It forms an integral part of various essential enzyme reactions in the body. If given in high dosage, it will cause the blood-serum cholesterol level to be lowered. A deficiency will result in the disease called pellagra, symptoms of which are a reddish skin rash of the exposed skin areas and diarrhea. Nicotinic acid deficiency can cause various mental changes such as irritability, anxiety, and depression, and its use has been shown to cause improvement in the emotionally disturbed.

Pyridoxine (B_6) appears in egg yolk, meat, fish, milk, whole grains, cabbage, and legumes. Necessary to several different reactions involving the body's building blocks, it has been called the amino-acid metabolism vitamin. Shortages are particularly obvious in infants who have irritability and convulsions. Deficiency symptoms in adults are similar to those in niacin and riboflavin deficiency, and include a greasy dermatitis in the eyebrows and at the angles of the mouth. Late symptoms are severe nervous disturbances and kidney stones.

Vitamin C is contained in citrus fruits, tomatoes, green leafy vegetables, potatoes, beans, asparagus, cabbage, turnips, cantaloupe, and strawberries. The best sources are uncooked. The biochemical action of vitamin C is poorly understood, but the results of its deficiency are readily identified clinically as a tendency for hemorrhage of the small blood-vessel capillaries of the mouth, skin, and covering of the bones with delayed wound healing. Vitamin C acts in some unknown way in protecting the body against infections. Recently, there has been a widespread supposition that it is effective against the common cold. This vitamin influences the absorption of iron from the intestines and, therefore, lack of it may result in anemia. Severe lack of vitamin C results in scurvy, in which the entire complex of the above symptoms are present.

Vitamin D is present in cod-liver oil, the flesh of oily fish (sardines, salmon, and herring), egg yolks, and liver. Sunlight will cause Vitamin-D precursors in the oily lubricating materials of the skin to be converted to vitamin D. It aids in promoting the absorption of calcium and phosphorus in the small intestine. Severe Vitamin-D deficiency can result in rickets, where the bones become soft and pliable, causing various deformities such as bowlegs, knock-knees, enlargements at the ends of the bones, and a narrow, distorted chest with beading of the ribs and contracted pelvis—all of which usually occur in childhood. Shortage may also result in symptoms associated with low-blood-serum calcium, some of which are leg cramps and irritability of the muscles. Adequate vitamin D is necessary for the maintenance of the bones and teeth.

Vitamin E occurs naturally in wheat-germ oil, peanut germ, corn germ, vegetable oils, eggs, milk, liver, and green leafy vegetables, and in a mixture of compounds called tocopherols. The biochemical function of vitamin E relates to its activity as an antioxidant for vitamin A and unsaturated fats. It helps prevent the latter from becoming abnormal peroxidized fats, which are toxic to the liver. Recently, it has been indicated that deficiency of vitamin E may increase the risk of a heart attack. There has been no definite clinical syndrome related to Vitamin-E deficiency but it has been used therapeutically in conditions such as muscular dystrophy, habitual miscarriages, multiple sclerosis, sterility, and menopausal conditions. The results obtained have been inconclusive, as they cannot be evaluated in a cause-and-effect relationship.

Vitamin B_{12}—beef liver and kidney are the richest sources. It is also found in good supply in muscle meat, eggs, milk, and cheese. There is no vitamin B_{12} in plant products. It performs in conjunction with what is called the "intrinsic factor" present in the stomach, the two being necessary for the formation of red blood cells. Lack of this vitamin, or the intrinsic factor, results in pernicious anemia. Normally associated with this is a deficiency of hydrochloric acid in the stomach.

Vitamin K is found in cabbage, cauliflower, kale, spinach, other green vegetables, tomatoes, cheese, egg yolk, soybean oil, and liver, and alfalfa is the richest source known. For vitamin K to be absorbed, bile is necessary. This vitamin is essential in the formation of a compound called prothrombin, which is a required component in the clotting of blood. A deficiency will cause internal hemorrhages, and minor wounds or slight bruises may result in extensive bleeding beneath the skin. In severe deficiency, blood may appear in the urine due to bleeding from the internal lining of the bladder.

Minerals

The human machine requires certain minerals. The more important ones are calcium, phosphorus, iron, iodine, magnesium, zinc, sodium, and potassium.

Calcium is an important constituent of all living cells and is present in very large quantities in bones and teeth. It is essential for normal heart action, muscle tone, nerve transmission, and blood clotting. Normal calcium concentrations in the blood will help prevent the porous destruction of bone structure, a condition called osteoporosis. Milk, cheese, and green leafy vegetables are the best sources of calcium, though it is also found in broccoli, baked beans, legumes, dried figs, dates, and eggs. Lack of calcium can cause muscle cramps and bone destruction.

Phosphorus is essential to the development of bones and teeth. It is part of several enzymes essential for the oxidation of foodstuff. Rich sources of phosphorus are meat, fish, eggs, milk, nuts, legumes, and whole grains.

Iron is vital to hemoglobin formation in the red cells of the blood and is found in all body cells, for it serves to transport oxygen to the tissue and to activate cell functions. Good reservoirs of iron are whole grains, egg yolk, beef (particularly beef liver), lean meats, legumes, nuts, fruits, and green vegetables. Anemia results from iron deficiency. In periods of demand for nutrition such as pregnancy and lactation and growth from infancy through adolescence, additional iron in the diet is called for.

Iodine combines with this protein tyrosine to form the thyroid hormone thyroxin. The best source is seafood such as salmon, cod, halibut, lobster, oysters, and kelp. Lack of iodine may cause goiter and lessening of thyroxin, the thyroid hormone. A relative lack of thyroid hormone lowers the metabolism and causes puffiness, lethargy, easy weight gain, and water-logged tissues and decreases the body's ability to burn fat as energy.

Magnesium is an important activator of several enzyme systems involved in nerve conduction. It is relatively abundant in vegetable greens. Deficiency of magnesium may result in increased irritability of the nerves and increased muscular contractibility, and finally in convulsions when a severe deficiency exists. Other symptoms of severe magnesium deficiency are mental disorientation, confusion, and hallucinations.

Zinc is a trace mineral and is necessary for growth and sexual maturation. It is a constituent of insulin. A deficiency of zinc is noted in children subsisting on diets high in cereals but low in animal products. Zinc occurs in animal and plant tissues in somewhat lesser amounts than iron.

Sodium is necessary for the vital fluid balance of our bodies, but excess sodium intake will cause water retention. This mineral is contained in table salt, bread, margarine; meats such as ham, bacon, corned beef, salt pork, and sausage; cheese, canned corn, peas, asparagus, and salted nuts. Symptoms of acute lack of salt include nausea, dizziness, muscular cramps, and mental apathy. Lack of salt is brought about by excessive sweating, vomiting, and diarrhea.

Potassium is a very important mineral, the lack of which brings extreme muscle weakness, lethargy, loss of appetite, weakness of the heart muscle, and distention of the intestines. Good, natural sources of potassium are orange juice, tomato juice, bananas, dried prunes, whole-wheat bread and whole-wheat cereals, broccoli, sweet potatoes, and oatmeal. Patients receiving diuretics should be sure to eat good portions of the above foods.

Nitrogen is the essential element for combination with amino acids to form the building blocks of all vital body cells. In growth periods, the body takes on nitrogen in combination with amino acids in new-formed cells and is said to be in positive nitrogen balance. In starvation and wasting diseases, cells are broken down and the freed nitrogen is excreted via the kidneys, causing negative nitrogen balance. Measurement of non-protein nitrogen in the blood serum yields a ready estimate of kidney function.

Fiber

This is the food element that adds bulk to your diet. It is found in fruit and in low-carbohydrate vegetables such as lettuce, asparagus, green beans, cabbage, celery, and squash. Fiber is necessary in the diet to help prevent constipation. *Fiber diminishes body fat storage by lessening the post-prandial glycemic effect of carbohydrates.*

Water

Many people who are dieting avoid drinking water because they want to lose "weight." Remember, we want to restore the internal body machinery and tune its working parts to efficiency. *I recommend that you drink six to eight glasses of water each day* since approximately two quarts of water per day are eliminated via the kidneys carrying off unwanted metabolic waste materials. Water is an essential part of the blood, lymph, and various secretions of the body, including the digestive juices. Water is the common solution wherein the many chemical reactions vital to health take place in the body. It is essential in the formation of fluids that lubricate our joints and it allows the intestines to move freely and efficiently in the performance of their functions within the abdomen. Water is the cooling fluid in the body, being evaporated from the lungs and skin surfaces. Without water, we could not exist for more than a few days. Relative lack of water causes a drying of the stool with resultant constipation and a lessening of the digestive juices, contributing to gas and bloating, and will tend to promote the accumulation of metabolic waste products, leaving us with a tired feeling and loss of body vitality.

If your heart and kidneys are functioning normally, and you do not ingest excessive salt, you will not hold water under normal circumstances.

Drink water—it is one of the good things in life that are free. If you want to improve its taste, add decaffeinated coffee, weak tea, or sugar-free flavorings. We will elaborate on this in chapter 8.

To Sum Up

1. You are protein. All body structures, including the glands, hormones, and enzymes, are composed mainly of protein amino acids.
2. Almost all of the body cells and hormones contain cholesterol and certain essential fats in their structure.
3. Protein and fat deficiency in the diet causes body inefficiency.

4. The body does not store protein as such, but only in the form of vital tissues, which can be broken down and changed to sugar (glucose) during dietary abstinence.

5. Fish and vegetable oils contain a much higher percentage of unsaturated than saturated fat.

6. Free fatty acid is the source of aerobic energy for the muscles. It is derived from stored body fat.

7. All carbohydrates are assimilated as blood sugar (glucose). Excessive carbohydrate ingestion causes insulin secretion by the pancreas and the storage of body fat.

8. The nervous system is a mandatory user of blood sugar (glucose) as its energy and this is maintained during dietary abstinence at homeostatic levels by conversion of tissue proteins to glucose.

9. Body fat cannot be converted into glucose. Once body fat, always body fat, until it is oxidized as aerobic energy by the muscles and other vital lean tissue.

10. The average Americans ingest far too many carbohydrates and not enough proteins and fats.

11. If we select properly from the wide variety of dairy, meat, fish, poultry, vegetables, and fruits, a balance of vitamins should be obtained.

12. Vitamin deficiency can result in many maladies.

13. In undernourished obese people, daily vitamin supplements may be necessary.

Chapter IV

What Happens to the Food You Eat?

The foods you eat are reduced to pulp by your teeth, moistened and lubricated by your saliva, and then passed into the digestive tract (Figure B). The three basic types of foods (fats, proteins, carbohydrates) are digested and assimilated by different methods and at different sites in the digestive tract, but in general, each type is digested and prepared for assimilation by protein compounds called enzymes.

The Carbohydrates

These, the sugars and starches, are first acted upon by the digestive enzyme ptyalin in the salivary juice of the mouth. This is a very good reason for chewing the carbohydrates thoroughly and allowing them to remain in your mouth for a moment before swallowing them. *The stomach acid has little effect upon the carbohydrates;* they are mainly digested in the small intestine by the enzymes, maltase, and amylase, which are present in the juices secreted by the pancreas. After absorption, the carbohydrates become blood sugar and are carried to the liver by the intestinal veins known as the portal system. They are transported via the blood to the brain and nerves to be used as aerobic energy and stored in the muscle as secondary energy. The brain is an obligatory user of glucose as its energy. However, the muscles store glucose as glycogen where it serves as a "reserve" anaerobic energy to be utilized in states where available oxygen is insufficient due to prolonged rapid and strenuous exercises. Stored muscle glucose (glycogen) cannot be liberated back into the blood. The liver is the only storage depot for sugar (glucose) that the brain can utilize.

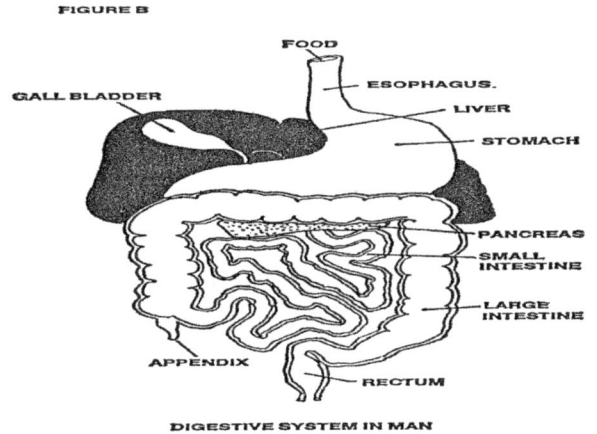

FIGURE B

FOOD

ESOPHAGUS.

GALL BLADDER

LIVER

STOMACH

PANCREAS

SMALL INTESTINE

LARGE INTESTINE

APPENDIX

RECTUM

DIGESTIVE SYSTEM IN MAN

The liver is the pivot point for all carbohydrate metabolism; in fact, *if the liver of an animal is removed, it will die within a period of hours*. Blood-glucose levels must be maintained at all times to continue the existence of the brain and nervous system, and in the absence of the liver, the body is unable to synthesize glucose from protein.

Fats

These are digested in the small intestine by the enzyme of the pancreatic juice, lipase, which acts in conjunction with the bile, secreted from the gallbladder. The ingested fats are absorbed by intestinal lacteals and pass into the lymph system to move via the thoracic duct, a large lymph channel that empties into the great veins at the base of the neck area. Absorbed fat thus bypasses the liver and passes directly into the bloodstream, where it is picked up in very small globules called chylomicrons. A major percentage of ingested fat eventually becomes the source of aerobic energy for the muscles and other vital tissues and raw material for cellular structure. That free fatty acid is the source of aerobic energy for the muscles, including the heart muscle, is a relatively newly established fact of biochemical research. It has been long established that almost all body cells contain fat molecules that are an integral and indispensable part of the cell structural makeup.

Proteins

First acted upon in the stomach by a bath of hydrochloric acid and by the digestive enzyme pepsin, they are further broken down in the small intestine by the digestive enzymes trypsin and chymotrypsin, which are secreted in the pancreatic juices. The end products of protein hydrolysis are the amino acids, which are absorbed into the veins of the small intestine and pass to the liver via the portal veins. In the liver, the amino acids are involved in various biochemical processes wherein they are synthesized into new protein molecules or are broken down and transformed into sugar by the liver in the process of gluconeogenesis. From the liver, they are carried in the bloodstream to the cells of the vital tissues, where they are synthesized into structural components of the cell.

In the liver, dietary protein or proteins derived from destroyed body tissues are converted into sugar (glucose) for those most demanding energy collectors, the brain and the nervous system. Aside from energy, the proteins are the essential elements of all the enzymes and hormones of the body and act as the critical structural element in every body cell.

Burning Up Fat

Clearly, eating food is not enough. It must be digested and assimilated. Some people have digestive-enzyme deficiencies. In that case, they can take the missing enzymes by mouth; physicians can prescribe them. The lack of digestive enzymes is recognized by symptoms such as bloating, dyspepsia, gas, and nausea.

For a better understanding of what happens to the food you eat, let's return again to the analogy of the automobile.

We all know that if a car is to work properly, all of its parts must be functioning efficiently—carburetor adjusted, valves ground, plugs cleaned, timing set, and the entire engine tuned up to its peak of performance. Likewise, the parts of the body—liver, kidney, heart, lungs, intestines, and glands, and so on—must perform at their peak if we are to burn up our excess fat.

Thus, the amount of fat we lose is determined not only by the food we eat but also by what our bodies do with it.

When fat is burned as energy, it is oxidized into carbon dioxide and water.

Some people have a "Cadillac engine," or are high oxidizers. Some people have a "Volkswagen engine," or are low oxidizers. A Cadillac engine will burn far more gasoline than will a Volkswagen engine. The parts that make up these engines determine how much gasoline is oxidized in combustion as fuel. The difference between the body's parts and the auto's parts is that the cells that make up the body parts are constantly being broken down and replaced with new cells. To keep the entire organ functioning at peak performance and peak fat consumption, a daily intake of proteins and certain fats is essential in the diet since these are the raw materials from which the cells of the vital body "engine" are made.

If you remember that the muscles and other vital body parts burn fat as aerobic energy, it becomes clear that when low-caloric regimens deficient in necessary proteins and fat cause our body "engine" to lose vital lean tissues, the result is an "engine" with less "horsepower" burning less of our unwanted stored body fat.

Animal studies have revealed that a starved animal may lose as much as 20 percent of its liver within the first two days of starvation. Although there are no human experiments specifically correlating this animal experiment, it can be safely concluded that *the liver in humans is mutilated similarly during starvation*, since it has been established by radioactively tagged isotopes that *over 50 percent of the weight loss in starvation is vital lean tissue.*

The average American diet is relatively high in carbohydrates and lacking in fat and protein. A relative protein deficiency tends to cause the body to hold water, while excess carbohydrates will increase body fat. This combination of eating excess carbohydrates and little protein will promote weight increase doubly, both by water retention and accumulation of body fat.

Fat-Reducing Diet

I believe that the *ideal diet for reducing body fat should approximate the diabetic diet; proportionately higher in protein and fat, and low in carbohydrate.* With this combination, the myriad needs for body cells, hormones, and enzymes from protein amino acids and the essential fatty acids are supplied, and the proteins needed to maintain blood sugar to the brain and nerves during fasting hours are provided. A low-carbohydrate intake will supply the initial blood sugar needed by the brain, nervous system, and certain enzyme systems. Keeping the carbohydrate intake low prevents the transformation of blood sugar to body-fat. Ingested fat will supply ready energy in the form of free fatty acids to prime the muscles to action and to burn more body fat while supplying a substratum for the essential structural elements in the vital cells and hormones of the body. More about your diet in subsequent chapters.

Diet and Constipation

Many overweight people are plagued with the problem of constipation. After the nutrients of our food have been digested and absorbed, the remaining undigested materials with accumulated wastes pass into the lower large intestine. The peristaltic movement of the large bowel then propels this waste material toward eventual disposal. The stimulus to the large bowel is stretching, and it is a fiber found in coarse green vegetables such as celery, cabbage, lettuce, and carrots and in fruit that supplies the necessary bulk to stimulate bowel action and help prevent constipation. Sufficient lubrication is also necessary, and this is assured by adequate water intake—six to eight glasses per day.

Fat Metabolism Studies

One of the most important works in biochemistry had taken place within the field of fat metabolism when the research team at Harvard won the Nobel Prize in Medicine in 1964 for their continued efforts in this area. Most people are still not aware of the full impact that this and other advances will have in the field of nutrition in the coming years.

The latest biochemistry and endocrinology textbooks have been rewritten in the sections concerning the way in which our bodies metabolize fat, and in the relationship of carbohydrate metabolism to fat metabolism. The *electrifying discovery that the fat cell, long considered an inert storage depot, is really a dynamic cell capable of changing blood sugar into body fat, has motivated work and progress at research laboratories throughout the nation* and may well change the current concepts about diabetes and coronary heart disease as well as previous thinking concerning nutrition and obesity.

A simple way to approach the new concept regarding fat metabolism is with a study of the *fat cell itself* (Figure C). The illustration of a fat globule shows how the fat cells appear in the subcutaneous tissue of the body. Remember, there are literally countless millions of these cells in your body. Though highly difficult to imagine, it has been established that at the thin cell membrane of the fat cell, there occurs a whole spectrum of metabolic and enzymatic actions that are involved in the transformation of blood sugar into fatty acids. If alpha-glycerophosphate, a metabolite of blood sugar, and insulin are available, the fatty acids manufactured form blood sugar or the fatty acids derived from the fat we eat are then stored in the central cavity of the fat cell as triglyceride, which contains three fatty acids combined with glycerol. The stored fatty acids in the triglycerides are the "gasoline" for the body and are released from the fat cell as free fatty acids upon energy demand by the muscles and other organs of the body. Glycerol, a trihybrid alcohol, is also released from the fat cell and is returned to the liver where it is transformed into glucose. However, this partial conversion of glycerol to glucose represents only a small fraction and is not sufficient to offset the conversion of protein to glucose during fasting states.

The best way I can describe the fat cell is to call it a balloon with a button on the side. The balloon itself is the fat-cell membrane, the button on the side is the nucleus, and inside the balloon is the stored fat. When fat comes out of the "balloons," they shrink in size and the person gets thinner. If fat goes into the fat cells, the "balloons" expand and the person gets fatter.

Recently, it has been established *that obese patients may have over three times as many fat cells as do thin people.* Fat cells evolve from primitive leptocytes, which mature into adult fat cells as the person becomes obese. This process begins in infancy. Therefore, people who are obese, with their much greater number of fat cells, have a greater capacity to store fat than would a thin person since, again, each fat cell is a fat factory capable of manufacturing and storing fat.

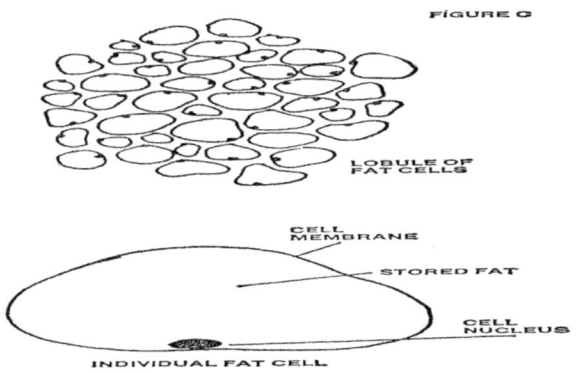

FIGURE G

LOBULE OF FAT CELLS

CELL MEMBRANE

STORED FAT

CELL NUCLEUS

INDIVIDUAL FAT CELL

High-Fat, Low-Carbohydrate Diets

One major key to the understanding of obesity is the knowledge that alpha-glycerophosphate, a glucose metabolite, and insulin must be available before fat can be stored in the fat cell. This is why people on high-fat, low-carbohydrate diets lose fat instead of gaining it.

When alpha-glycerophosphate and insulin are not available, ingested fat is carried to the muscles to be used as aerobic energy, and increasing the metabolic rate, causes more of the stored fat to be oxidized and lost. Fat is either going into or coming out of the eon millions of fat-cell balloons. When carbohydrates, the major blood-sugar precursors, are not available, there is little chance of fat production and storage.

The metabolic and enzymatic activities occurring in the fat cell were previously thought to take place only in the liver. Consequently, the thinking about nutrition, with regard to the capacity of the body to change sugar (glucose) to fat, was thus oriented. Previous thinking that fatty acids stored in the fat cell could be reconverted to sugar (glucose) led to the *fallacious idea that sugar (glucose) was the main energy source of the body*. We now know that glucose is the mandatory energy for the brain and nerves, but is a secondary energy of the muscles.

To Sum Up

1. Your food is digested by enzymes, the lack of which prevents its assimilation and causes indigestion.
2. All carbohydrates become blood sugar (glucose) after digestion and assimilation.
3. During fasting intervals, proteins are converted to glucose in the liver, which maintains blood-sugar levels in the brain and nerves.

4. Excess carbohydrates are changed to fat at the fat-cell membrane of each of the countless millions of fat cells in the body.

5. The fat cell, long considered an inert storage depot, has acquired a new and startling identity. We now know it to be an active cell capable of complex biochemical reactions that promote the conversion of blood sugar (glucose) to body fat.

6. There can be no storage of body fat without alpha-glycerophosphate, a metabolite of blood sugar and insulin secreted by the pancreas when the blood sugar rises.

7. The quality, quantity, and frequency of the meals are critical factors in planning a body fat reduction and lean tissue maintenance diet.

Chapter V

Glands And Hormones

The Endocrine Glands

The hormone-producing glands abstract cholesterol and essential fatty and amino acids from the bloodstream from which the hormones are synthesized. They are then secreted directly back into the blood according to the body's demands. These glands are ductless and are called endocrine glands in contrast to glands with ducts such as the salivary glands, which are known as exocrine glands.

The endocrine glands serve as the regulators that keep the magnificent internal biochemical machinery of your body functioning in an orderly manner and allow its adaptation to an almost infinite variety of circumstances and conditions. Their position in the body can be more easily understood if illustrated (Figure D).

The Pituitary Gland

It has been called the body's master gland since it secretes a variety of hormone substances that regulate the life-sustaining secretions of other hormone-producing glands. They were given the name trophin, meaning of or pertaining to nutrition, and they are secreted mainly in the anterior portion of the pituitary gland.

The anterior pituitary adrenocorticotropic hormone regulates the secretion of the adrenal glands and is active during emotional stress. The thyrotropic hormone regulates the secretion of the thyroid gland. The gonadotropic hormone regulates the secretions of the sex glands. And the growth hormone regulates the degree of growth from infancy to maturity.

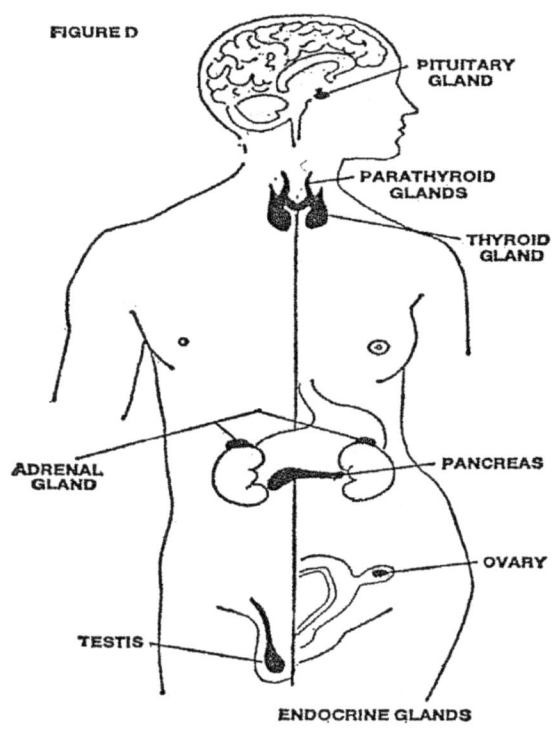

FIGURE D

PITUITARY GLAND

PARATHYROID GLANDS

THYROID GLAND

ADRENAL GLAND

PANCREAS

OVARY

TESTIS

ENDOCRINE GLANDS

In 1965, a new hormone called lipotropic was isolated at the University of California. Lipotropic, it was learned, *causes stored body fat to be released into the bloodstream, where it is transported and then oxidized as energy by the muscles* and other vital tissue. Though not generally available to physicians in its purified form, it may prove to be a substantial help in the future for the treatment of obesity.

The posterior portion of the pituitary secretes two hormones, vasopressin and oxytocin. Vasopressin is commonly called the antidiuretic hormone, because, in its absence, large volumes of water may be passed. Excess antidiuretic hormone will cause fluid retention.

Oxytocin assists in the secretion of milk by the nursing mother and instigates uterine contractions during childbirth.

The Thyroid Gland

The many actions of the thyroid's hormone, thyroxin, have not been clearly established, but in general, thyroxin accelerates the metabolic activity of all body cells.

It will increase the circulation by dilating the blood vessels to some extent and by stimulating the heart action. It helps maintain gamma globulin, the protein used by the body in fighting disease. Thyroxin also increases the absorption of sugar from the intestinal tract into the bloodstream; thus people lacking thyroxin may have low blood sugar. Thyroxin is a necessary hormone for efficient action of the gonadal hormones, and slow or underdeveloped sexual maturation may result when this hormone is deficient. Numerous clinical findings associated with thyroid deficiency include susceptibility to infection, dry skin, coarse and brittle hair, loss of hair, flaky fingernails, skin eczemas, edema or water in the tissues, apathy, mental depression, and lack of sexual interest.

Regarding obesity, it is generally believed today that the thyroid hormone has a role in the breaking up of stored fat present as triglyceride into free fatty acid used as an aerobic energy source by the muscles. It will increase the production of alpha-glycerophosphate dehydrogenase, which, by inactivating alpha-glycerophosphate, will cause a decrease in fat production and storage in the fat cell. By increasing the general metabolic rate, thyroxin causes more free fatty acid to be oxidized as energy by the muscles, resulting in an increased loss of unwanted body fat.

The Adrenal Glands

These cap the kidneys bilaterally, each gland having two compartments, the cortex and the medulla. The adrenal cortex secretes hormones generally classified as corticoids, one of which is hydrocortisone, performing a wide range of important actions. It is the anti-inflammatory and anti-allergy hormone, effective in reducing reactions caused by allergies, arthritis, asthma, and severe stress.

Aldosterone is secreted by the adrenal cortex and causes the kidneys to retain sodium, resulting in the accumulation of intracellular fluids in the body.

Adrenal male sex hormones, androgens, are also produced by the adrenal cortex. These, if secreted in excess in the female will cause such secondary male sex characteristics as facial hair, excess hair on the abdomen and pubic area, and enlargement of the clitoris.

The adrenal medulla, the other major division of the adrenal glands, secretes adrenalin. Adrenalin constricts the small arteries of the intestinal circulation, opens the heart and muscle arteries, increases heart action, and opens the bronchial tubes of the lungs. *Adrenalin can also cause an increase in the release of stored liver glycogen and glucose, which subsequently supplies an immediate source of energy to the brain and nervous system.* It similarly causes the liberation of free fatty acids from the fat cells, thus furnishing the muscles with an instant source of aerobic energy.

The Pancreas

Situated in the lap of the first part of the small intestine, the duodenum, the pancreas secretes several digestive enzymes as described in chapter 3, but its main hormone is insulin. For years, it was stated that the action of insulin was that of increasing the use of glucose by the cells, for it was assumed that the sole source of energy to the entire body was sugar (glucose). We know now that the main action of insulin is to change excess blood sugar into body fat, and that the *main source of energy to the muscles and the vital lean tissues is not sugar (glucose), but fat*—sugar being the mandatory energy source to the brain, nervous system, and germinal layers of the gonads. Insulin is necessary too for the limited storage of glucose as glycogen in the muscles which acts as a secondary source of energy to the muscles when available oxygen is insufficient.

Insulin also discourages the fatty acids within the fat-cell sphere from entering the bloodstream to be used as energy. *It thus prevents the body from losing fat. Clearly then, insulin is the major villain concerning obesity.* It is a double-barreled gun—not only does it cause fat production and storage, but it prevents us from losing body fat. Insulin is secreted whenever the blood sugar rises above normal limits. All carbohydrates are digested and assimilated as blood sugar.

But the pancreas secretes another hormone called glucagon, and very recent research indicates that *glucagon acts antagonistically to insulin.*

The ratio between insulin and glucagon determines whether the liver will dump glycogen, stored glucose, into the bloodstream. The net effect of excess glucagon as compared to insulin is to elevate the blood sugar. A thus unrecognized cause of diabetes may be related to an excess of glucagon rather than a deficiency of insulin.

The Reproductive Glands

These are the testes in the male and the ovaries in the female. The testes elaborate the hormone testosterone, which promotes the development of the sex organ and secondary sex characteristics of the male. It causes the growth of facial hair, abdominal and pubic hair, and enlargement of the penis and vocal cords resulting in the lower pitch and resonance of the male voice. It may increase sexual desire in both sexes, but its use as an aphrodisiac is ill-advised, particularly in the female, because she might develop secondary masculine sex characteristics.

Testosterone is a necessary hormone for the utilization of the building blocks of the cells, the amino acids, and to increase the size and the strength of muscles. Testosterone deficiency in the male may result in "feminine" distribution of body fat, with increased deposition about the buttocks and hips and overdevelopment of the male breasts.

The ovaries secrete the female sex hormones, estrogen and progesterone. Estrogen is responsible for the development of secondary sex characteristics in the female—growth of underarm and pubic hair, enlargement of the breast, and the general feminine distribution of fat. It also aids in the repair of the womb lining after menstruation. Lack of estrogen may lead to irregular menstruation and underdeveloped breasts. In menopause, this lack causes the symptoms of "hot flashes," thought to result from periodic stimulation of the adrenal glands by the pituitary gland in the absence of the female hormones. Lack of estrogen can result also in the destruction of the inner matrix of the bones, resulting in osteoporosis.

Progesterone, the other female hormone, prepares the lining of the womb for implantation of the fertilized egg and also maintains the lining during pregnancy. It has some diuretic effect, causing a loss of body fluid. This hormone is produced by the ovary at about midway in the menstrual cycle. Clinical uses of progesterone have prevented miscarriages and assisted obese patients who show an ovarian deficiency with fluid retention.

The Parathyroid Glands

These help to maintain the calcium ion level in the blood. This is important because calcium in normal concentrations affects the contractibility of the heart and skeletal muscles of the body and maintains the integrity of the bones.

To Sum Up

1. Recently, a pituitary hormone called lipotropic has been isolated, the main property of which is to send stored fat into the bloodstream to be burned as energy.

2. Thyroid hormone is thought to assist in sending stored fat as fatty acid, the aerobic energy source to muscles as well as to the heart. It increases the general metabolic rate and therefore indirectly causes more fat to be lost. It also assists in reducing body fat storage.

3. Aldosterone, an adrenal hormone, causes water retention.

4. Insulin causes excess blood sugar (glucose) to be converted to fat and also tends to discourage the loss of body fat.

5. Prolonged therapy with estrogens may cause fluid retention and subsequent weight gain.

6. The antidiuretic hormone of the pituitary gland, vasopressin, causes water retention. Obese patients may have excess antidiuretic hormone.

7. Adrenalin will promote immediately available energies causing a rise in blood sugar, energy to the

brain and nerves, and free fatty-acid, the aerobic energy to the muscles.

8. Excessive adrenal output can cause secondary masculine sex characteristics in the female.

9. Lack of testosterone can cause a feminine fat distribution in the male.

Chapter VI

Hormones as Related to Obesity

Knowledge of the glands, and the hormone products they manufacture, has been a fascinating and continuous study throughout the history of medicine, but only during the recent past have major advances been made in revealing the action and interrelationships between glands. Many new techniques have assisted this advance. We now have the osmometer, an instrument that measures the electrolyte concentrations in body fluids in a matter of minutes. Various modes of color analysis called chromatography have revolutionized the analysis of amino acids, fatty acids, and other biochemical compounds. Ultraviolet and infrared spectroscopy have permitted new analyses of proteins, enzymes, and other substances. Even though tremendous strides have been made in the field of biochemical and endocrinological medicine, it is still in the early stages of its development. Undoubtedly, future accomplishments will further illuminate the inner workings of our body machinery, possibly to an un-dreamed-of state of sophistication.

Hormones and Fat Metabolism

For years, we have observed how some people can eat large amounts without gaining weight, while others eat very little yet do gain. The conclusion has been that there must be something wrong with their glands. This analysis may have been more accurate than anyone really realized. There are several products of the glands that have a direct effect upon fat metabolism. We have learned how insulin is responsible for the conversion of blood sugar (glucose) to fat, therefore tending to promote obesity, and how thyroid hormone increases the rate at which fatty acids are burned, therefore rending to stimulate body fat loss.

Many other glandular substances, active in the promotion of body reactions, aid the loss of stored body fat. These hormone substances promote the release of free fatty acids from fat cells into the bloodstream, where it serves as aerobic energy power to the muscles, including the heart. They are: (I) the adrenocorticotropic hormone of the pituitary; (2) cortisone from the adrenal glands; (3) the growth hormone of the pituitary; (4) adrenalin from the adrenal glands; and (5) a recently isolated hormone called lipotropic, which is also a pituitary-gland secretion.

Weight Gain from Hormonal Imbalance

Although the direct effect of these hormones may be the loss of body fat, the total effect occasionally may induce a gain in that ambiguous item "weight," usually due to water retention. This is particularly significant in the person who may be secreting a relative excess of adrenocorticotropic hormone because of emotional anxiety. In anxiety, this pituitary hormone will induce secretion of cortisone from the adrenal glands, changing proteins into glucose, and dumping stored glucose from the liver into the bloodstream, with subsequent rising of serum glucose levels. *The chronically anxiety-ridden and overactive person, if a female, will many times have an unwanted fat ridge on the thigh* about ten inches below the hip joint, and will exhibit *very firm tissue due to accumulation of intracellular fluid.* This is thought to be the result of periodic over activity of the pituitary gland, cortisone secretion, and elevated blood sugar, bringing on an excess secretion of insulin with subsequent fat storage. These people have great difficulty in losing body fat.

If the pituitary fails to secrete tropic hormones—due to exhaustion after years of overactivity or tumor encroachment—a kind of obesity will occur where the body fat is flabby and redundant and distributed like the body fat in a thyroid deficiency. Other factors are loss of secondary sexual characteristics—lessening of the breasts, lack of under-arm and pubic hair, and relative reduction of the sexual organs with decreased potency and low blood sugar.

Most women suffering a relative ovarian deficiency show excess fat on the hips above the hip joint and may be deficient in the breast area. Patients with thyroid deficiency are obese, lethargic, have water-logged tissues; have dry skin and coarse, brittle hair; and have elevated serum cholesterol. Their facial appearance is characteristically puffy and the body fat is distributed in a trunk fashion, with body measurements of chest, abdomen, and hips being in close approximation.

Keeping Insulin Production Down

Only during recent years has the medical profession come to realize that insulin is the hormone necessary to produce and store body fat. In fact, it can be safely said that if you were devoid of insulin, you would have very little fat on your body. On the surface, this appears contradictory, since for years it was held that most diabetics were deficient in insulin. We now know that most obese diabetics have developed insulin resistance due to the increased sizes of the distended fat cells and subsequently have increased serum insulin levels.

Insulin not only causes us to gain more fat, but it will also discourage fat loss. Therefore, insulin secretion by the pancreas must be discouraged. This is done by preventing the blood sugar from rising above normal limits. Insulin is secreted by the pancreas when blood sugar rises above normal limits.

Leptin

The fat cells produce leptin, a hormone that acts in the appetite center of the brain to decrease the appetite for sugar. Leptin is released by the fat cells in concert with the release of insulin, the fat-storing hormone of the pancreas. As the storage of triglyceride (fat) within the fat cell continues, the fat cells expand. Over time, the resulting stretching of the fat cell membrane increases the resistance of the fat cell to the fat-storing action of insulin. The subsequently continued elevation of the blood sugar will promote an increased release of leptin from the fat cell which, *when in excess*, decreases the sensitivity of the brain's appetite center to leptin. Most obese people have high serum levels of both leptin and insulin. Restricting dietary sugars and starches to breakfast and eating more healthy fats will lower both serum leptin and insulin levels. Lowering serum leptin levels will increase the brain's sensitivity to leptin and therefore curb the appetite for sugar. Lowering the serum insulin level will decrease the storage of body fat, the primary goal in the treatment of obesity.

Diagnosing Hormonal Imbalance

In briefly viewing the hormones and glands in the last two chapters, it readily can be seen that the endocrine system is vastly complex, and the action and interaction of the hormones in regulating body function is a marvel, indeed. We have seen how excess insulin or a relative lack of thyroid hormone tends to promote obesity and how other hormones discourage it.

The proper balance of body hormones is the highest goal to be sought. Either excess or deficiency will cause a condition of hormonal imbalance.

I believe that there are literally thousands of undiagnosed cases of borderline deficiencies or excesses of specific hormones.

Recently a condition referred to as the hypometabolic syndrome, or a state of decreased metabolism, has been recognized wherein patients exhibit easy weight gain, easy fatigability, depression, and dry skin with some degree of facial puffiness. Yet, the thyroid-function rests fall within the "normal" range. We still have much to learn in this area of Bariatrics—a new medical specialty.

In general, it may be held that improper nutrition, failure to provide the necessary nutritional foundations for the synthesis of body hormones, and psychological factors play an important role in causing glandular functional imbalance. Any specific treatment regarding glandular imbalances is, of course, within the realm of your physician.

Of late, a new field of medicine has emerged, the science of bariatrics. Bariatrics is derived from the Greek word *baros*, meaning weight. Bariatricians are physicians who specialize in treating obesity. Loosely labeled "fat doctors," the great majority of these physicians are dedicated men with special knowledge and experience in the fields of nutrition, endocrinology, and internal medicine, which are all integrally related to the problem of obesity. They realize that just cutting calories is not the answer, but rather a total approach, which includes the latest knowledge in the sciences of medicine and nutrition.

Glands and The Nervous System

The main parts of the nervous system are the brain, spinal cord, and nerves. The voluntary nervous network is involved in consciousness and mental efforts, as in speech, vision, hearing, taste, touch, and muscular behavior. Contrarily, the involuntary nervous system regulates our various internal organs, such as the salivary glands, heart, lungs, stomach, intestine, liver, gallbladder, pancreas, adrenal glands, rectum, bladder, kidneys, and sexual organs. All these organs are involuntarily affected by two distinct families of nerves, sympathetic and parasympathetic. Generally, sympathetic nerves are activated in emergency or stressful predicaments, the parasympathetic nerves acting as regulators during normal activity. Wonderfully, one system counterbalances the other.

Many glands are stimulated by nerves. Thus it is that emotional and/or critical situations affect the secretions of our glands. Research is showing increasing evidence that the two systems, nervous and glandular, are inter-related.

Recent anatomical research has discovered a circulation between the pituitary gland and the hypothalamus, the place of emotional origin and the appetite-control center in the brain. This is called a "portal circulation" and closely resembles the link existing between the liver and the intestines. It was so labeled because it is not a part of the general circulation, remaining instead an independent link between the emotional and appetite centers in the brain and the master pituitary gland which regulates the secretion of the other endocrine glands.

The two great communications systems of the body—nervous and glandular systems—are interrelated and function in a closely coordinated fashion.

To Sum Up

1. Though significant steps have been made, we still are in the embryonic phase in the study of hormone-producing glands.
2. Some glandular hormones that help discharge body fat are the pituitary's and adrenocorticotropie hormone, cortisone, thyroid, adrenalin, and lipotropic.

3. Glandular imbalance will promote certain distinct fat distribution, altering the body shape.

4. A relative thyroid deficiency is one cause of obesity.

5. Excess insulin activity results in body fat gain.

6. The majority of glandular imbalances have roots within emotional disturbances, improper eating habits, or systemic changes in the body.

7. The two great communication systems of the human body—endocrine and nervous—are interrelated.

Chapter VII

Psychological Aspects Of Obesity

Once aware that there is actually a direct anatomical relationship between the nervous and glandular systems, we can begin to fathom the basis for psychosomatic medicine. The psyche refers to the mind, the soma to the body. Psychological factors are an important influence on the cause and aggravation of many diseases, including obesity.

In contemplating the behavior of man as related to his eating habits, an understanding of the mental and emotional processes is very helpful. Behavior, almost without exception, is influenced by a person's basic needs, which are emotional, intellectual, and physiological.

Major emotional needs include love and affection, and a sense of belonging to the particular group with which one is identified.

An important intellectual need is self-expression, or the chance to portray to others the creative aspects of one's own personality. In today's culture, the general tendency is to conform to whatever the Joneses are doing—thus the basic need for self-expression is frustrated in countless examples. One must be very strong and resilient indeed to overcome the overriding influences toward conformity.

Central physiological needs are food, sex, and clothing and shelter. In this highly technical and accomplished society, many people are able to satisfy their basic physiological needs. But because of the very nature of today's accelerated world, they may not succeed in fulfilling their emotional needs, particularly in regard to love and affection. So pronounced in our society is the emphasis on sex that many people mistake sexual expression for love, thus neglecting the need for love with sex and leaving it unsatisfied.

Why People Overeat

If a basic intellectual or emotional need is frustrated, tension will result. Many frustrated people are eating compulsively to help alleviate such tensions, especially those persons who *during childhood were constantly gratified by food as a substitution for affection.* Carbohydrates, particularly "sweets," serve the majority of these compulsive eaters.

But this is obviously an age of uncertainty, and anxiety and tension are the logical results of many of our problems. The complexity of modern life, the dangers inherent in virtually all forms of modern transportation, the possibility of sickness, the concern for economic security, the threat of nuclear war, the basic continuing uncertainty about our origin and place in the universe, and our concern for the future—all these intangibles create tension and anxiety, which many attempt to discharge through overeating.

Beyond the external causes of tension, *many conflicts are created within.*

A person may have certain impulses or tendencies out of step with the established moral standards of his society. This too builds conflict, and all conflict results in tension and anxiety. Such a person may overeat to compensate for his failure to find peace.

Many are over-eating because of hostile feelings, some of which may be directed inwardly in a self-destructive tendency, the fulfillment of self-ruin being represented by the acquisition of excess body fat.

Psychological Conditioning

Another very important factor that causes people to overeat is simply *what they think about*. We are highly influenced by what we are exposed to via communications media. *The unending bombardment of glamorous carbohydrate-food advertisements strongly affects our thinking*, and a great many people respond to these ads by altering their eating habits.

Advertising is simply a form of conditioning wherein a person is conditioned to think about products—food and all else—to the extent that he will act upon this conditioning and purchase the particular product involved. Food ads are especially alluring.

In a culture blessed with an overabundance of food, beautifully packaged, endorsed, advertised—and this culture being tense and uncertainly directed—it's inevitable that one of the main preoccupations of its people is food. Another is sex. And when purveyed to the public in the same way food is, sex, like food, becomes a mass-escape item.

Along with the positive conditioning to overeat, there is also a definite negative conditioning that brings the same result. Strangely, this is taking place through *the culture's strong emphasis on being and remaining slender* in the face of multitudinous pressures urging people to eat. The resulting conflict also produces anxiety. In many instances, the actual pressure to evade eating may contribute to a person's rebellion and subsequent gratification by overeating. The method I propose in this book solves this dilemma since the person must eat three meals and two between-meal snacks a day and no food is entirely disallowed.

Calorie counting is actually a form of indirect negative conditioning, since every time we count and consciously limit our food intake, we are impressing on our subconscious the word "food." This practice leads a person to be perpetually engrossed by the thoughts of food but with the admonition "Don't eat it!" Again, we have a *source of conflict* with likely rebellion and overeating.

Auto-Suggestion

The same psychological principle of conditioning can be used to help us avoid overeating and improper eating habits. One excellent method is that of *auto-suggestion*.

Auto-suggestion is an excellent approach available to anyone. This practice is receiving wide popularity and is a takeoff from Coué, who popularized the method in the 1920s. You may have seen or heard the phrase: "Every day in every way, I am getting better and better." To some, this may sound a bit silly, but actually, it's a very concrete method of influencing the powerful subconscious mind, which plagues many people but could become their greatest asset. Applying this to obesity, one might daily affirm to his subconscious mind: "You will overcome your bad eating habits. You will eat three nutritious meals and two between-meal snacks a day containing proteins and essential fats. You will not eat carbohydrates between meals. You will become trim, healthy, and attractive."

The actual wording of these daily affirmations may be altered; but the idea is to repetitively employ effective directions to the subconscious mind, by which your goal of becoming trim and attractive will become a reality.

It has been said that what we become is determined by the thoughts we entertain. *Many obese people are defeating their own purpose because of negative thoughts, hostility being the primary one.* They have a good reason for being hostile. It's not easy to feel rejected and unwanted. It's not easy to feel uncomfortable in public. However, our thoughts can be controlled. Maybe we have not been aware of our hostile feelings and resulting attitudes, which may cause others to reject us. I am sure most of us don't realize that in many instances, we are eating the "wrong" foods because of our hostile feelings and are expressing this hostility by hurting ourselves. We can't seem to strike back at others, so it's our own selves we strike at by putting on more of that ugly unwanted fat.

Thousands today are afraid; they fear the word fat and all of its connotations. So many times what we fear will materialize. Rather than letting fear grow, use your creative imagination to "see" in your mind the image of that attractive, slender individual you have always desired to be.

Think of yourself as being that person, as acting, moving about, eating as that strong and slender person does. Think thin. Much more about obtaining a slender and attractive body image using self-hypnosis in Chapter XI.

Demonstrate the courage to take those positive steps that will reverse any negative and defeatist attitude you may have, and enable you to overcome your obese condition once and for all. Substitute positive thoughts and reinforce them with daily affirmations: "I am becoming thin. I will overcome." And never, never become discouraged.

Of course, to achieve desired results, the primary requisite is that you truly wish to. Because of negative psychological attitudes such as hostility and fear, many obese people are defeating their own purpose. These negative attitudes may be expressed by eating just those things that you know you shouldn't. Understanding the problem will go a long way toward reversing these negative attitudes. Once you firmly grasp the fundamental principles of what your food is—why you should eat more of the proteins and certain fats but avoid excessive carbohydrates—you are already halfway toward achieving the desired results.

Substitute positive thoughts for negative ones. Visualize yourself becoming trim and attractive. This is a much more accurate goal than "losing pounds."

The power of thought is a mighty one, and we can become the masters of our thinking or we can let others think for us. Too many today are doing the latter. Far too many have been told to "lose weight" by cutting calories. Replace that slogan with "eat more of the right foods" but restrict the wrong food to breakfast in order to regain and maintain vital tissues in muscle, kidney, liver, etc., and in time, rid yourself of your unwanted coat of fat."

Words are the tools of thought. Everyone has been urged to use the tools "resist," "stop eating," "push yourself away from the table." Resisting is a negation of something and can become tiring and end in capitulation.

The correct mental tool to use is choice. Choose the right foods, at the right time, in the right amounts. It will surprise you how much easier and less-tiring choosing is than is resisting. More about what, how much of what, when, and how often you should choose appears in the next chapter.

To Sum Up

1. Frustrated psychological needs can cause undesirable eating habits.

2. Advertising affects our thinking through conditioning and may contribute to improper eating habits.

3. Calorie counting may become a negative conditioning practice and may contribute to overeating.

4. Auto-suggestion is an excellent way to enforce good eating habits.

5. Our thoughts determine what we are. Positive thinking and using imagination to "see" our new image is a very helpful method of obtaining desired results.

6. Thinking before eating by choosing the right food is the positive way of obtaining proper eating habits.

Chapter VIII

The QQF Lifetime Way of Eating

It seems that this is the diet-craze age. Have you tried the grapefruit diet? "Mayo Clinic" diet? Egg diet? Soup diet? High-protein diet? Starvation diet? Etcetera, etcetera. To say that we have been confused by the plethora of diets would be an understatement. Here we will attempt to clarify matters by discarding the word "diet" and replacing it with the phrase "a way to eat" since your first objective in solving your problem is to understand that you must eat to lose. Do I detect a note of skepticism in your reaction? Eat to lose? Yes—and you must also think before you eat.

What Kind Of Food Is What?

In Chapter 3, an understanding of what the food you eat is, what it does, and why it is necessary for good health was given. Let's review this briefly again because an understanding of, and ability to recognize the kinds of food you are eating, is a major key to your problem.

Essentially, there are three kinds of foods: proteins, fats, and carbohydrates. An easy way to recognize proteins is to ask yourself the question, "Did this food come from an animal source?" Eggs, meat, fish, fowl, and cheese are all from animal sources and are excellent protein foods. Most animal sources also contain fat.

Fats? They include olive oil, canola oil, corn oil, and other vegetable oils, the omega-3 fish oils, butter, and the fat in fish and meat. There are also many hidden fats and their percentages are listed in Table II of chapter 3.

Carbohydrates? These are: (1) sweets—candy, pie, cake, soft drinks, ice cream, rolls, and pastries, all made from refined sugar and high in carbohydrates, and natural sugars contained in all fruits; and (2) starches—bread, macaroni, and spaghetti and vegetable such as peas, corn, potatoes, and lima beans, all having high percentages of carbohydrates. The exact carbohydrate contents of most common food can be found in your Never After Breakfast Carb Counter in the appendix.

The thought processes involved in recognizing the different kinds of food will enable you to be selective in your shopping at the grocery store and in choosing more intelligently from a menu when dining out.

Think About What You Eat

Now, what to choose? How much to choose? And when to choose it? These questions involve you and the solution to your problem. I will try to answer them as we go along, but you must seek out the answers too and apply them to develop the eating habits necessary to become trim and attractive.

Even if you did know what, how much, and when, you might find yourself asking the question: Why don't I choose? As we have seen, there are many psychological factors involved that contribute to compulsive overeating, and here, I believe, is a major reason why so many obese people are overeating, and many without even realizing the food is in their mouths. It is simply that they do not think consciously of what they are doing. *Thinking before eating* is a major key to your problem.

One woman told me that she rarely enjoyed her food even in the best of restaurants. She always ate very rapidly. On one occasion, her husband interrupted her while she was busily chewing away and talking and asked her, "What are you doing?" With that, she began to think about the wonderful filet mignon she had been ingesting, and to her amazement, for the first time experienced the savor and flavor of an expensive steak already half consumed. If you will hesitate ten seconds before you eat, and think about what you are about to do—to eat—and then concentrate on what you are eating while chewing, I am sure you will be surprised to find real enjoyment and pleasure in eating and be satisfied with less.

So many people have lost their enjoyment because of another condition, "dietitis," worrying about eating anything for fear they will gain "weight." If nothing else, I want you to know that your enjoyment of eating need not be subdued any longer. In fact, again, you must eat to lose, *to lose fat.*

The Correct Approach to Dieting

Let's examine the diet that will help you accomplish the wonderful results, a slender figure together with better health, more vitality, and greater attractiveness.

During the past several decades, there have been revolutionary breakthroughs in the field of metabolic research. Key breakthrough information, upon which this new way of eating and losing body fat is based, is:

1. Every fat cell of the body—there are billions—is a miniature fat factory.
2. Ingested fat cannot be stored as body fat without the blood-sugar (glucose) metabolite called alpha glycerophosphate and without insulin, secreted by the pancreas, when the blood sugar rises. (All carbohydrates are digested and assimilated in the body as blood sugar [glucose].)
3. Ingested carbohydrates can be changed into and stored as body fat at the fat-cell membranes of the billions of fat cells in your body fat.
4. Your body fat cannot be re-converted to the blood sugar needed at all times by the brain, nervous system, and germinal layers of the gonads. In dietary abstinence, the proteins in muscles, liver, blood, kidneys, and other organs are broken down and converted to blood sugar.
5. Up to 60 percent of the weight lost in starvation is vital tissues from muscle and other lean tissues, not fat.
6. Fat in the form of free fatty acids, not sugar (glucose), is the major aerobic energy source of the

muscles and of other vital lean tissues including the heart.

7. Vegetable oils added to a low carbohydrate diet may increase the oxidation and loss of excess body fat by 20 to 25 percent.

With these key breakthrough points in mind, let us examine the specific goals to be accomplished by this diet:

1. We want to stop gaining any more body fat. This is done by preventing insulin secretion by controlling the blood sugar. Since all carbohydrates are assimilated as blood sugar, these are restricted in this diet.

2. We want to lose the excess fat we have already accumulated. This is done by increasing the metabolism by eating more of the vegetable oils and fat-containing proteins and by daily physical exercise.

3. We want to regain and restore lost vital tissue, which may be due to severe and prolonged caloric restriction. This is done by eating complete proteins and essential fats that the body cannot manufacture.

4. We want to lose excess body water. This is promoted by reducing salt in the diet and by drinking more water, six to eight glasses every day.

This diet, or way of eating, *in general, can be classified as high in fat, moderate in protein, and low in carbohydrates.*

Dr. Edgar Gordon of the University of Wisconsin, in the *Journal of the American Medical Association*, October 1963, published a similar diet, which I have modified and added to as a result of extensive study and over forty years of clinical experience treating obese patients. Having been highly disillusioned with the caloric-restriction method, I sought out and found a better way, which is presented in this book.

Dr. Herman Taller, in his book *Calories Don't Count*, advocated the restriction of carbohydrates and ingestion of vegetable oils at a time when key information was not yet available to the medical profession, and consequently his views were not enthusiastically received. Other unfortunate circumstances led to a general disregard and even condemnation of his valuable contribution, which I consider a tragedy. Dr. Taller was on the right track and will no doubt be recognized as a pioneer in the field of obesity treatment. Dr. Robert Atkins has published several books in which he has advocated the ketogenic diet by restricting daily carbohydrates to 20 grams and allowing a gradual increase but with strict and continued restriction. In his book, *Dr. Atkins' New Diet Revolution,* Dr. Atkins stated that there are two major energies of the body: ketones and glucose. The major aerobic energy to the muscles, including the heart, is fat as free fatty acid. Glucose is the mandatory energy to the brain and nerves and the secondary energy to the muscles. Ketones are a reserve energy, formed in the liver during states of extreme deprivation of dietary carbohydrates which may be used to a limited extent by the brain.

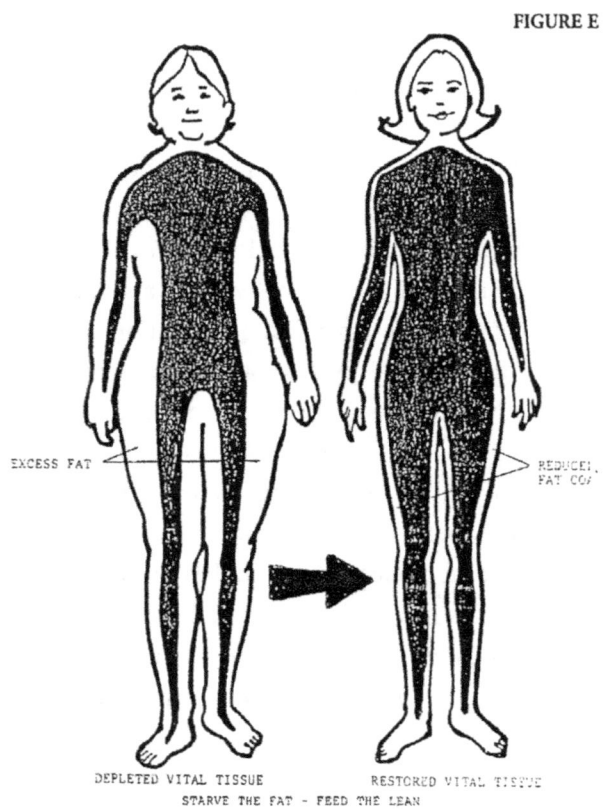

EXCESS FAT

REDUCED
FAT CO/

DEPLETED VITAL TISSUE   RESTORED VITAL TISSUE
STARVE THE FAT - FEED THE LEAN

Most people dieting by the caloric-restriction method have been avoiding the high-calorie protein-plus-fat foods (the leanest meat contains fat) and have been eating excessive amounts of sugars and starches. Many eat only one meal a day. As a result, they have become depleted of muscle and other vital body tissues and in actuality have become a thin person under a heavy coat of fat. I am convinced that a diet reversal—eating more fats and proteins and fewer sugars and starches—will replenish the essential body structure and reduce the carbohydrate-induced fat coat. (See Figure E.) Since ingested fat is a ready source of muscle energy and is an essential nutrient in body cellular and hormone structure, I strongly advocate an adequate intake of essential fats in the diet in a ratio of two unsaturated to one saturated. (See Table II, chapter 3, for relative percentages of saturated and unsaturated fats.)

As we pointed out before, the term "weight" is grossly general, since weight can be lost or gained in any of three body components as vital tissues, body fat, or water. Similarly, the term "fat" is a gross generalization, actually a "scare" word implanted over the years through such severe brain-washing that some people entirely avoid avocados and butter and eat little or none of the vegetable oils. People should understand that certain fats are an essential part of your diet. Fat cannot be defined as a single item since there are many variations of fatty-acid molecules for which our bodies have a real need.

What About Carbohydrates?

Some of my patients, previous to be being treated, had tried to avoid carbohydrates entirely. This is wrong, as the liver storage for sugar is limited to between 50-75 grams, and therefore severely restricting carbohydrates will cause a condition called ketosis after this supply is depleted. Ketosis results from the formation of ketone bodies in the liver. Ketones are a limited reserve energy source for the brain. A moderate degree of ketosis for short periods may aid the loss of body fat, but extreme ketone-body accumulation is harmful since it will cause acidosis which in diabetics can be fatal. Keeping the daily carbohydrate intake over 30 grams will prevent ketosis and promote fat loss.

My Prescribed Diet

I sometimes explain this diet to the patients by the analogy of the fireplace. When you rise in the morning in a cold room, you build a fire with paper, cardboard, wood, and logs. The same holds for the body. Upon rising you should eat a good breakfast to "warm up" your body. The sugar and starches are the paper, and the proteins and fats are the logs and wood.

Eating the sweets at breakfast will cause your empty liver supply to be refilled with sugar (glucose). The proteins and fats serve as a continuing energy source to maintain both sugar and fat energy levels until the noon meal.

The ideal way to eat is to recognize the foods on your plate for what they are. This can make eating very interesting, very pleasurable. The proteins are easy to remember if we associate them with meat, fish, fowl, eggs, and cheese (complete animal proteins) and complete vegetable proteins found in yeast, soybeans, and wheat and corn germ. "Incomplete" vegetable proteins are found in grain cereals, beans, wheat, and peas. The most obvious fats are the oils, butter, and the visible fat on meat. And remember, most meat, fish, and fowl proteins contain a good percentage of fat regardless of how "lean" it is. It almost seems that Nature has wrapped the protein package in fat since it's difficult to find a tasty protein that does not contain fat. *Daily ingestion of fat is advised*, to provide a substratum for lean-tissue synthesis and to increase the burning and loss of your stored body fat. As stated before, it should be taken in a ratio of two unsaturated to one saturated. Sugars, "sweets," and fruits are restricted to breakfast. Vegetable and grain carbohydrates are limited by gram count and are to be eaten in moderation at the noon and evening meals and at breakfast if desired.

Although of major importance, carbohydrate counting is only one aspect of this diet and the total caloric intake per day is not of major importance. The proportion of carbohydrates, fats, and proteins at each meal, the number of meals, and the time sequence of food ingestion are all important. It's what, how much of what, when, and how often—not just how much you eat—that counts. *You must eat three meals per day,* ceasing each meal when you feel well-nourished and alert, but *avoiding any stuffed, full feeling.* Protein and fat snacks are encouraged between meals. This will prevent *any desire to indulge in carbs between meals.* A listing of desirable between-meal snacks is provided in the appendix.

Breakfast is the most important meal of the day and it is here that sugar-containing foods such as fruits, fruit juice, cinnamon rolls, pie, and even cake are encouraged in moderation. *After breakfast, all sweets, fruits, or refined starches and caffeine are to be avoided.* In general, you should avoid foods containing refined starches and refined sugars, but by all means, restrict the refined sugars to breakfast. *During the day, such sugar-containing foods as candy, cake, pie, soft drinks, and fruit are absolutely forbidden,* since they will cause the blood sugar to rise, insulin to be secreted by the pancreas, and thus cause you to gain more body fat.

It is interesting to note that New Englanders have been eating pie for breakfast since the first Thanksgiving Day. In Greece, you will find coffee and rolls and honey served at breakfast, but very few if any pastries served at the noon and evening meals, where oils are substituted for the sweets.

At breakfast, you may have salt, sweets, fruit, fruit juices and drink coffee, but after breakfast, substitutes may be advised; for sugars, nuts; for coffee, decaffeinated coffee. (I'll explain this a little further along.) Use salt in moderation. In hot weather, you may use more salt on your food.

Each meal is to contain a goodly portion of animal protein—eggs, meat, fish, chicken or cheese. A suggested amount of meat or fish is 3-5 ounces. Here one might ask, *"How does a vegetarian maintain good health?"* A knowledgeable vegetarian, if ingesting a proper balance of grain and vegetable proteins, may be able to supply the eight essential amino acids (those that the body cannot manufacture) in a complete package and at one time, necessary to synthesize new body tissue. This would be difficult, to my way of thinking, and therefore I recommend the animal-source proteins, which always contain the essential eight amino acids. Even here, seek a variety among the meat, fowl, dairy, and fish proteins.

A fresh salad of greens is to be eaten at the noon and evening meals well saturated with two or three tablespoons of the vegetable oils such as corn oil, safflower oil, canola oil, olive oil, or soybean oil because these oils *increase your metabolism and cause you to burn more of your unwanted body fat.* If you will eat butter and saturated fat at breakfast and the unsaturated oils at the noon and evening meals, the ratio of one saturated to two unsaturated is fostered. This has been devised as an optimal ratio to *assure the intake of essential fats vital to the structural elements of the body cells and hormones.*

Many people make the mistake of dieting by skipping breakfast, snacking for lunch, then eating ravenously at supper and on into the evening. This technique is the worst possible method of dieting because it will promote sarcopenic obesity where depleted muscles and other lean tissues are covered with excessive layers of body fat. More about the significance of sarcopenic obesity later on.

Don't Count Calories

A good rule of thumb for knowing how many calories to consume is to avoid any feelings of fullness when completing your meal. And don't be hungry when you finish eating, but rather feel well-nourished and alert. The daily caloric need of any individual will vary according to his state of nutrition, the climate, and the amount of physical exercise in which he engages. It is much more logical to *allow your body needs to dictate when you've had enough food rather than set an arbitrary caloric limit—you should be satisfied, well-nourished and alert after finishing your meal.* One excellent way to assure that you do not go on compulsively into caloric excess is to always leave something on your plate, even if it's a scrap of bread. This habit will act as a psychological "red light" and stop you from compulsively continuing to eat too much. Try it, it really works.

If your physician feels that, though overweight, you are suffering from malnutrition in the form of vital-tissue depletion, you will have to eat more proteins and fats than others should, and he may advise that *you snack on meat or fish between meals.* As you regain vital tissue, you will note less sagging of tissue and a restoration to a feeling of more vitality and energy. Between-meal consumption of sugar, caffeine, in fact all carbohydrates, is prohibited regardless of your state of protein nutrition because they only cause you to gain more body fat.

Keep the Diet Discipline

To become habitual, any system depends upon regular observance. To avoid rebellion, eat between-meal protein-fat snacks every day.

Allowable between-meal snacks are a teaspoon of peanut butter right from the jar, pork rinds, sardines, nuts, i.e., almonds, and chicken livers. etc., A complete list of between-meal snacks may be found in the appendix. For those who further wish to diminish their appetite between meals, I advise emptying a packet of unsweetened gelatin into a glass of water and drinking the contents slowly.

After a period of one or two months eating three meals and two between-meal snacks every day, a desire for sugars diminishes to the extent that a small piece of chocolate between meals may equal the experience of eating two or three or even four pieces. *If your plate contains protein and fat at each meal, you will likewise be surprised to find you have less desire to eat a large meal.* On the other hand, if your meal is predominantly carbohydrate, you are apt to continue eating, and leave the table feeling unsatisfied. This appears to be the nature of the carbohydrates—they do not satisfy and often actually increase the appetite.

A fair proportion for each meal is 80 percent fat and protein, 20 percent carbohydrate. At breakfast, the percentage of carbohydrates is higher because after the overnight fast, carbs are needed to restore the supply of glycogen in the liver. We will amplify this critically important factor in Chapter IX.

These "Ten Commandments" sum up the method of dieting recommended:

1. You must eat 3 meals a day. No need to count calories. Finish your meal feeling well-nourished and satisfied, but never "full" or hungry.

2. Eat complete proteins at each meal, 3-5 ounces of meat, fish, or fowl, 1-2 ounces of cheese or 1-2 eggs daily. Have fish 3-5 times a week. (See pg. 125-127 for a list of complete proteins)

3. At breakfast, eat any food you like. Up to 30 grams of carbohydrates are allowed. A daily vitamin-mineral supplement is recommended at breakfast.

4. Refined sugars, i.e., sweets, cake, pie, cookies, and candy, etc.; refined starches, i.e., white bread, biscuits, bagel, muffins, and other high glycemic carbs; fruit juices; sugar and caffeine-containing drinks, i.e., coffee, tea, or cola drinks, are to be completely avoided after breakfast. See the Never After Breakfast Carb Counter in the appendix.

5. At the noon and evening meal raw, steamed or cooked vegetables are recommended for their vitamin, mineral, and fiber content. Low glycemic carbs are limited at the noon and evening meals. Take 2-3 tbsp. of MCT[1] oil, olive oil, canola oil, corn oil or safflower oil on a green salad or in a bowl of soup.

6. You may have between-meal protein and fat-containing snacks, i.e., pork rinds, beef jerky, a small piece of cheese, olives, or nuts as desired. See the appendix for a list of between-meal snacks. Avoid all carbohydrates between meals.

7. Drink more liquids, 6-8 8-oz. glasses of water per day. Sugar and caffeine-free diet drinks, decaffeinated coffee, herbal tea, or Aloe Vera juice are allowed as desired.

8. Use salt sparingly on your food. Other seasonings, i.e., oregano, thyme, black or white pepper, horseradish, garlic, etc., are allowed as desired.

9. In general, choose natural foods, i.e., fresh fruits, raw vegetables, whole wheat bread, cereals, grains, legumes, cheese, lean meat, fish or fowl, and vegetable oils over processed foods. Certain processed foods are desired, i.e., MCT oil (fractionated coconut oil) and tofu (soybean curd).

10. Think Thin. See the image of that trim and healthy person you've always wanted to be in your mind's

---

[1] MCT oils, medium chain triglycerides, enter the liver via the portal vein. Hence, they avoid the general circulation and are less likely to be stored as body fat.

eye, and keep it there until it becomes a reality. You can become trim and attractive if you think you can.

For Best Results

This method should be considered as a life-time way of eating that will enable you to nourish your body and rid yourself of unwanted excess body fat. If properly enforced, it can achieve the desired results in a large percentage of overweight people who are in normal health. Those obese people who follow this diet conscientiously, but do not lose weight or measurements, should seek the help of their doctor since diet may not be enough. Their problem likely lies in a biochemical or glandular imbalance within the body. And of course, anyone suffering from an ulcer, from kidney, heart, gallbladder, or liver disease, from gout or from other medical conditions, must be under the direct supervision of a physician.

It can be seen from the sample diets, outlined on pages 109-119, that each meal provides an adequate supply of protein and fat, and the carbohydrates have been restricted, up to 30 grams at breakfast and between 15-20 grams at the noon and evening meals. The typical daily meal plan will often exceed 1,000 calories, but remember *the quality or kind of food is the critical factor, not the number of calories.* Once again, it's the QQF: the quality, quantity, and frequency; it's what, how much of what, when, and how often—not just how much you eat—that counts.

This dietary approach offers very wide latitude in the selection of food and is relatively simple since all sugars and refined starches are restricted to breakfast. Most protein and fatty foods are very low in carbohydrates and thus, for all practical purposes, can be overlooked with regard to counting their carbohydrate value.

One of my goals was to devise *a diet that did not require continual referral to tables*. The best results appear once a person becomes familiar with the proteins and fats, which need not be counted. In the beginning, reference to the carbohydrate chart will be necessary to ascertain the exact gram content of any particular food, but the more common items will be easily remembered after a short period.

Exchange methods have been used in the past wherein the total calorie intake is limited as well as the type of food being eaten, similar to the exchange diets used for diabetic patients. In these diet plans, foods are divided into six groups: milk, bread, meat, fat, fruit, and vegetables. The patient may select exchange items from each list, which is regulated by the total number of calories to which the person is restricted. I believe this method to be somewhat cumbersome, for it demands constant reference to tables, which might invite rebellion in certain patients. The great benefit of this way of eating is that there are no absolute no-no's and no food is taken away from you. There will be no compulsions to fall off the wagon. Therefore, you will be able to stay with this new way of eating, lose excess body fat, restore your vital tissues and maintain a trim and attractive body.

Your diet provides a proper food balance of nutrients, vitamins, and minerals to restore vital body tissue and does not exceed the carbohydrate limit necessary to prevent body-fat production.

In 1981, Dr. David Jenkins of the University of Toronto developed the glycemic index, a rating comparing the glycemic effect (producing the rise in serum glucose of various carbohydrates after digestion) to the glycemic effect of pure glucose. This rating system is a definite improvement over the traditional division of carbohydrates into simple sugars with a greater glycemic effect than complex starches. However, the clinical value of the glycemic index is limited since serving sizes vary and the glycemic index of many carbohydrate-containing foods has not yet been determined. Sugars, fruits, and refined starches have higher glycemic values and are restricted to breakfast whereas most of all vegetables have a lower glycemic value and are encouraged at the noon and evening meals. The general division of sugars and starches to those eaten only at breakfast and those allowed at any meal is a clear and effective way to keep blood sugar and insulin levels lowered and consequently to prevent the storage of body fat.

Many overweight patients have subsisted on an unbalanced diet for many months—perhaps even years—and thus present themselves to their physician in a state of malnutrition, suffering from various deficiencies. From an adequate dietary history, the physician can estimate the existing deficiency or deficiencies and can establish treatment as to diet and medication.

Beverages

Sugar-free, calorie-free, and caffeine-free beverages are permitted as desired. Many of my patients wonder why they cannot drink black coffee after breakfast. It has been demonstrated that caffeine promotes insulin secretion by the pancreas, which will induce fat production. Caffeine has been restricted for years in diets for patients who demonstrate insulin over-activity. While it is true that many thin people drink excessive amounts of coffee, they are undoubtedly oxidizing fat as energy as fast as it is produced. The obese person cannot afford to store any added fat. Cola drinks, diet or otherwise, contain caffeine and are therefore restricted to breakfast.

The suggested daily menus on pages 109-119 indicate the wide variety of foods that can be eaten under this dietary plan. A number of the lunch and dinner meals may not contain vegetable oil. *Following any lunch or supper that does not include vegetable oil, 1-2 omega-3 oil capsules may be taken after the meal. This will help increase the metabolic rate, and therefore increase the "burning" and loss of your unwanted fat.* A daily supplement of 400-800 units of Vitamin-E is recommended while taking vegetable and fish oils.

Sample Daily Diet Outline

Suggested Breakfast

*Fruit, juice, milk

*Muffins, biscuits, whole-wheat bread with honey or preserves, butter, pastries

*1-2 egg yolks

*Bacon, sausage, ham, fish, 1 cup of coffee with cream

Breakfast is the time to please the palate. You may eat anything you desire.

After breakfast, self-discipline is the way of life. Eat only the staples—meat, fish, poultry, cheese, oils, vegetables, grains. All fruits, sugar, refined starches and caffeine-containing foods are to be absolutely avoided.

Suggested Lunches

*Tossed green salad with lettuce, tomatoes, and onion, 2-3 tablespoons of vegetable oil with vinegar

*Meat pie, hamburger, tuna, sardines, salmon, other animal protein

*½ slice of whole-wheat bread with soft margarine or butter

*Carrots or celery

*1 cup of decaffeinated coffee with cream

Suggested Dinners

*Tossed green salad with 2-3 tablespoons of vegetable oil and vinegar

*Asparagus, cauliflower, artichoke, green beans, other low-carbohydrate vegetables

*Steak, fish, chops, chicken, cheese, other animal protein, ½ slice of whole-wheat bread with soft margarine or butter, 1 cup of decaffeinated coffee with cream

Suggested Between-Meal Snacks

*Almonds, pork rinds, beef jerky, olives, oysters, crisp bacon, etc., (See Appendix for a complete listing)

* choice of

Note:

1. Limit carbohydrates (vegetables, fruits, sugars, and starches)—eat up to 30 grams at breakfast and 15-20 grams at the noon and evening meals.
2. Animal proteins (meat, fish, fowl) are not counted for carbohydrate content.
3. No fruit, sugar, refined starches, or caffeine after breakfast.
4. Between meals, eat no carbohydrates; protein and fat-containing snacks are allowed.
5. Finish each meal feeling nourished and alert and never be hungry after each meal.

Suggested Daily Menu #1 (Monday)

BREAKFAST		Grams
Grapefruit	½ raw with salt	14.0

Cheese omelet	1 egg	3.0
Grated cheese	¼ cup	
Rye toast	1 slice	12.0
Whipped butter	1-2 pats	trace
Coffee with cream	1 cup	0.0
		29.0

LUNCH

Avocado	½ medium	6.0
Shrimp, canned	½ cup	1.0
French dressing	1 tablespoon	3.0
Whole-wheat bread	½ slice	6.0
Soft margarine	1-2 pats	0.0
Decaffeinated coffee with cream	1 cup	0.0
		16.0

SUPPER

Tomato, sliced	¼ medium	1.8
Onion, green	1	0.9
Parsley, chopped	1 tablespoon	trace
Oil and vinegar dressing	3 tablespoon	0.7
Cracked-wheat bread with margarine	½ slice	6.0
Decaffeinated coffee with cream	1 cup	0.0
Bouillon soup	1 cup	0.0
T-bone steak, broiled	1 medium	0.0
Mushrooms, sautéed	½ cup canned	3.5
String beans	½ cup	3.0

Whole-wheat bread	½ slice	6.0
Butter	1-2 pat	0.0
Decaffeinated Coffee with cream	1 cup	0.0
		15.9

Suggested Daily Menu #2 (Tuesday)

BREAKFAST		Grams
Banana	½ medium	15.0
Scrambled egg topped with parsley	1 large	1.5
Bacon	1 slice crisp	trace
Whole-wheat toast	1 slice	12.0
Butter	1-2 pats	trace
Coffee	1 cup	2.0
Sugar and cream	½ tablespoon	
		30.5

LUNCH		
Coleslaw	½ cup	6.6
Fish sticks, breaded	2	3.0
American, cheddar or jack cheese	5 thin strips	0.5
Rye bread	½ slice	6.0
Butter	1 pat	trace
Decaffeinated Coffee with Cream	1 cup	0.0
		16.1

SUPPER

Iceberg lettuce	¼ head	3.5
Oil-and-vinegar dressing	3 tablespoons	0.7
Mashed potatoes	¼ cup	6.0
Butter	1-2 pats	
Ham	1 slice	0.0
Cracked-Wheat bread	½ slice	6.0
Margarine	1 pat	
Decaffeinated Coffee	1 cup	0.0
Cream		
		_____
		16.2

Suggested Daily Menu #3 (Wednesday)

BREAKFAST		Grams
Orange juice	½ cup	13.0
Breakfast steak	1 medium	0.0
Egg, any style	1 large	0.3
Whole-wheat toast	1 slice	12.0
Whipped butter	1 pat	trace
Coffee with cream, with ½ Sugar	1 cup ½ tsp	2.0
		_____
		27.3

LUNCH		
Broiled American cheese on a thick patty of ground beef	1 slice	0.6
Rye bread	1 slice	12.0

Lettuce leaves	4 large	1.0
Tomato slices	2 medium	2.0
Decaffeinated Coffee with Cream	1 cup	0.0
		15.6

SUPPER

Crabmeat cocktail	3 ounces, canned	1.2
Halibut steak, Broiled with garlic-and-butter sauce	medium size	0.6
Broccoli, Baked with grated Parmesan Cheese, Basted with Bouillon	1 cup	7.2
Whole-Wheat Bread	½ slice	6.0
Butter	1-2 pats	traces
Weak tea	1 cup	0.0
		15.0

Suggested Daily Menu #4 (Thursday)

BREAKFAST		Grams
Tomato juice	4 ounces	5.0
1 lamb patty	Medium	0.0
Egg, any style	1 large	0.6
Whole-Wheat Toast	1 slice	12.0
Grape jelly	2 teaspoon	10.0

Butter	1 pat	
Coffee with cream	1 cup	trace
		27.6

LUNCH

Hot corned beef or	2 slice	0.0
Pastrami with	½ cup	4.5
sauerkraut		
Rye bread	½ slice	6.0
Mustard	1 tablespoon	0.8
Tomato, sliced	½ medium	3.5
Dill pickle	1 small	1.5
Decaffeinated coffee	1 cup	0.0
with cream		
		16.3

SUPPER

Tossed green salad	14 cup	3.0
Oil-and-vinegar		1.0
dressing		
Chicken broth	1 cup	0.0
Broiled chicken	3-5 ounces	0.0
basted with chicken		
broth, mixed with		
lemon juice, and		
garlic powder		
String beans	1 cup	6.0
Baked potato	¼ small	5.3

Soft margarine	1 pat	0.0
Decaffeinated coffee with cream	1 cup	0.0
		15.3

Suggested Daily Menu #5 (Friday)

BREAKFAST		Grams
Apple	¼	5.5
Pancake, buckwheat	¼ inch-cake	10.7
Molasses, blackstrap	¾ tablespoon	8.2
Link sausages	2	0.0
Butter	2 pats	0.0
Tea, hot	1 cup	2.0
Sugar	½ tsp	
		26.4

LUNCH		
Iceberg lettuce	¼ head	3.5
Tomato wedges	1 medium	7.0
Oil-and-vinegar dressing	4 tablespoons	1.0
Steak, broiled	1 medium	0.0
French bread	½ slice	5.2
Soft margarine	1 pat	0.0
Decaffeinated Coffee with Cream	1 cup	0.0
		16.7

SUPER

Asparagus, green	6 spears	3.0
Mayonnaise, with lemon juice	2 tablespoons	trace
Leg of lamb, roast	slice	0.0
Mushroom soup	½ cup	10.2
Whole-wheat bread	¼ slice	3.0
Hot weak tea	1 cup	0.0
		16.2

Suggested Daily Menu #6 (Saturday)

BREAKFAST		Grams
Peach, with syrup pack	1	11.6
Poached egg with butter	1 large 1-2 pat	0.6
Bacon, crisp	2 slices	0.0
Rye toast	½ slice	6.0
Strawberry jam	2 teaspoons	9.4
Coffee with cream	1 cup	trace
		27.6

LUNCH		
Frankfurter (all-beef)	1 medium	2.0
Mustard	1 tablespoon	0.8
Chicken-noodle soup	¾ cup	6.5
Saltine crackers	2	6.0
		15.3

SUPPER

Carrot-Grated, raw	1 carrot	5.1
Mayonnaise	1 tablespoon	trace
Cottage Cheese	¼ cup	2.0
Hamburger Steak broiled	3-4 ounces	0.0
Baked Potato with	¼ small	5.0
Cheese Sauce	1 tablespoon	1.2
Whole-Wheat Bread	¼ slice	3.0
Soft margarine	2 pats	0.0
Decaffeinated coffee with cream	1 cup	0.0
		16.3

Suggested Daily Menu #7 (Sunday)

BREAKFAST		Grams
Doughnut, cake-type	½	8.0
Egg, fried	1 large	0.3
Pork sausage, patty	4 ounces	0.0
Biscuit	1	14.0
Butter	1 pat	0.0
Coffee with Cream	1 cup	2.0
or Sugar	½ tsp	
		24.3

LUNCH		
Tossed green salad		3.0
Oil-and-vinegar dressing	4 tablespoons	1.0

Tuna, canned, with mayonnaise and seasoning	3-4 ounces	0.0
Sweet Pickle	1 small	3.8
Tomato wedges	½ tomato	3.5
Rye bread	½ slice	6.0
Weak tea	1 cup	0.0
		17.3

SUPPER

Boston butter lettuce	¼ head	1.5
Chopped parsley	1 tablespoon	trace
Oil-and-vinegar dressing	4 tablespoons	1.6
Pork chop	1	0.0
Buttered Carrots	¼ cup	2.4
Brussels sprouts	¼ cup	2.0
Pumpernickel bread	½ slice	7.9
Soft margarine	1-2 pats	trace
Decaffeinated coffee with cream	1 cup	0.0
		15.4

Saccharin or other sugar-substitute-containing liquids are not recommended. The governmental ban on cyclamate-containing liquids and foods should cause you no alarm if you had been consuming these products. Experimental rats from birth were given cyclamate in amounts over fifty times the maximum recommended daily allowance for adult human beings for continuous and extended periods before cancers were noted in the rats' bladders.

You should drink 6-8 oz glasses of water per day to provide the necessary fluids so vital to the metabolic processes and promote the diuresis of accumulated body water.

A swallow of milk is helpful for allaying hunger in the evening prior to retiring and milk or cream may be taken at breakfast in your coffee or on cereal.

Alcoholic Beverages

These are allowed in moderation if they are not mixed with sugar-containing liquids. Recent research indicates that blood sugar may be expended through the metabolism of alcohol. And although alcohol does contain calories, by keeping alcohol and sugar separated they apparently are not stored as body fat. Although the "beer belly" (there are 14 grams of carbohydrate per bottle) is well known, whoever head of a "Bourbon belly?" In any event, do not drink alcohol at breakfast, your time to drink fruit juice.

Smoking

Many people smoke while drinking. Nicotine induces the transfer of free fatty acid from the fat cells into the bloodstream, and therefore reduces the appetite. This may explain why people experience weight loss when smoking. However, smoking is not recommended, because of the health hazards associated with prolonged cigarette use.

Appetite Suppressants

It has only recently been shown that the *main action of most so-called appetite-suppressant drugs is to promote lipolysis, to mobilize free fatty acid from the fat cells into the bloodstream.* Perhaps this is the reason they depress the appetite, for fat is an excellent appetite appeaser. Unfortunately, when taking these drugs in excess, people have also avoided eating proteins and fats, which results in vital tissue depletion. *This condition of depletion, in turn, "demands" nutrition, which may cause a return to random overeating and the regain of weight.* In place of drugs, the ingestion of vegetable oils will sustain fatty-acid levels in the bloodstream and hence will decrease the appetite between meals.

Remember, fats are satiating, whereas sugars and refined starches compel us to eat more. Eat more proteins and essential fats and restrict sugars and refined starches to breakfast. I know you will be happy and amazed at the results.

A Lesson from Animals

For years, farmers have used high-protein meals to put flesh on livestock. Hogs are fed high-protein content because hog producers want to sell ham, not fat. And hog buyers *will never buy a hog by its scale weight alone,* but always examine it to determine whether the animal is lacking muscle and is mostly fat-apparent from the general body contour. Life-insurance companies would do well to take a lesson from hog buyers. The Body Mass Index charts they publish should include ideal measurements as well, for specified heights and body weight.

People who raise horses know that eliminating the animal's starchy foods, feeding it a high protein-fat diet, and toning its muscles with daily exercise will create a beautiful form in a short while.

One can learn a great deal about nutrition by visiting the zoo. *Lean lions and tigers are fed several pounds of meat and fat, whereas the fat bear is fed a huge stack of bread, lettuce, apples, carrots and a small piece of meat.* In autumn to gain body fat, prior to hibernation, *the bear exists on a diet that is approximately 75 percent carbohydrates.* But, in spring, the bear goes to the river or lake for fish to rebuild muscle loss from hibernating during the long winter.

Restricting Carbohydrates

Since the body produces fat when our blood sugar and insulin levels become elevated, our precise goal of preventing more fat accumulation is to prevent the blood sugar from rising.

It can't be repeated too often—all carbohydrates are digested and assimilated as blood sugar. Ingesting sugar and refined starches will cause a sudden rise in blood sugar which causes insulin secretion by the pancreas. Body fat cannot be stored without insulin; therefore sugars and refined starches must be restricted to breakfast.

Our bodies have a check in this regard. In the lateral lining of the oral cavity, there are salivary glands with ducts that pour out juices called ptyalin. Whenever you eat carbohydrates, take small bites, chew them thoroughly, and allow them to mix momentarily with the digestive salivary juice before swallowing. I am convinced that this practice of chewing and thoroughly masticating the carbohydrate foods will limit the amount of them you will consume. The taste buds are located at the base of your tongue. Most enjoyment of eating disappears in the all-too-prevalent method of taking "steam-shovel" bites and dumping the food past the taste buds into the esophagus in large chunks. Too many of us are in a hurry. The old army slogan, "Hurry up and wait" is applicable to the manner in which many of us eat. We hurry the food into the stomach, eating too much in the process, and wait for that "full" feeling that tells us we are "satisfied." You will enjoy eating fruit, bread, and vegetables more if you will be careful to take smaller bites, chew thoroughly, and allow your food to mix with the salivary digestive juices in your mouth. This process is not as important with proteins and fats since they are digested lower down, in the stomach and the small intestine.

In general, all fruits contain high percentages of sugar (fructose). Vegetable starches high in carbohydrate are peas, corn, potatoes, and lima beans. White-sugar (sucrose) will cause sudden rises in blood sugar and is by all means restricted to breakfast.

Look at the table in the appendix at the back listing the carbohydrate-gram values[2]. Pick out the low numbers which will be very safe. However, don't forgo the large numbers entirely. For example, six stalks of asparagus came to only 3 grams—plenty of asparagus for anybody and entirely safe. One apple is 22 grams. This doesn't mean that you shouldn't eat any apples at all. Why not eat a quarter or half of an apple, and at breakfast? Simply take smaller bites, chew thoroughly, and allow the proper mixing with the

---

[2] The gram counts listed include the fiber content. Consequently, the carb count listed will have a lesser glycemic effect.

digestive juices in your mouth. I know that you will be pleasantly surprised to find the quarter or half of an apple eaten slowly more satisfying than a whole one gulped down.

Limiting carbohydrates will stop you from producing more body fat and allow you to lose your outer fat coat by burning it in the metabolic processes of your everyday activity and in planned physical exercise.

Balancing the Diet

Your other goal is to gain on the inside, the real you—muscle, kidneys, glands, liver, and other vital organs. These are composed of protein and essential fats. A variety in your intake of proteins and essential fats is necessary in order to achieve this. Balance your protein intake among the dairy, meat, fish, and poultry products, and select from vegetable and fish oils and from the wide variety of vegetables, fresh fruits, and grain products.

Many patients have told me they had entirely given up potatoes, for instance, because they are high in carbohydrates. Please understand that all foods are allowed and that no one food is to be entirely excluded. High-carbohydrate foods are counted, to be sure, but are not to be entirely eliminated from the diet, because a wide variety of foods is essential to assure a balanced dietary intake.

"Variety is the staff as well as the spice of life." One of my patients, a cook, used color in assuring a variety to her meal preparation. Her method was to form a nutritional mosaic by having always at least four different colors of the food on her table. This could be an aid to the housewife who wishes her family to have a healthy balanced dietary intake.

Green, leafy vegetables, red tomatoes, yellow squash, red and brown meat, white milk, and brown bread. Yes, color can be a real help to you in securing a balance in your eating habits.

In Table III are listed a selective variety of foods under the three general classifications of protein, fats, and carbohydrates.

Table III

COMPLETE PROTEINS
(Select one at each meal)

MEAT

Boiled Beef	Flank Steak	Smoked ham
Roast Beef	Beef Vegetable Stew	Pastrami
Corned Beef	Without Potatoes	Pork steak
Ground round, Chuck and Shoulder	Chipped Beef	Toast pork
	Filer Mignon	Pork chops
	Frankfurter	Rabbit
Dried Beef	Natural Unthickened Meat Juice	Salami
Beef Liver	for Gravy	Veal cutlet
T-Bone Steak		Veal chops
Rib Steak	Lamb Chops	Roasted veal
Porterhouse Steak	Roast Lamb	Venison
Pot Roast	Lamb Shoulder	Chili Con Carne

Round Steak	Baked Ham	Hungarian Goulash
Sirloin Steak	Boiled Ham	Meatballs
Swiss Steak	Fried Ham	Meatloaf

FOWL

Boiled Chicken	Chicken Liver	Broiled Quail
Broiled Chicken	Roasted Duck	Broiled or fried Squab
Canned Chicken	Roasted Pheasant	Roasted Turkey
Fried Chicken	Eggs	

SEAFOODS

Canned Abalone	Pike	Fried Scallops
Fried Abalone	Red Snapper	Boiled Shrimp
Anchovies	Lobster tail	Broiled Filet Sole
Catfish	Clams	Baked Fillet Sole
Pickled Herring	Baked Codfish	Broiled Whitefish
Broiled Lobster	Fried Bass	Fried Whitefish
Mackerel	Baked Bass	Fog Legs
Dried Oysters	Baked Haddock	Frozen Crab
Fried Oysters	Broiled Haddock	Fresh Crab
Fresh Oysters	Fried Halibut	Canned Crab
Oyster stew	Canned Sardines	Crabmeat Salad

Perch	Broiled Scallops	Broiled Salmon
Baked Salmon	Snails	Fried trout
Baked Swordfish	Baked Trout	
Smelt	Broiled Trout	

DAIRY

Milk
Cheese of all varieties

VEGETABLES

Soybeans
Wheat germ
Corn germ
Yeast

B. FATS
UNSATURATED OILS

Safflower oil	Corn oil	Soybean oil
Cottonseed oil	Peanut oil	Olive oil
Canola oil		

NUTS

Almonds	Cashews	Peanuts
Pistachios	Walnuts	

(See Appendix for a complete listing)

SALAD DRESSINGS

Oil and vinegar	French	Thousand Island
Mayonnaise	Roquefort	
(in moderation)		

C. CARBOHYDRATES
FRUITS
Moderate-High

Rhubarb	Cantaloupe	Cranberries
Gooseberries	Grapefruit	
Pineapple	Blackberries	Honeydew Melon
Loganberries	Pears	Cherries red, white, black
Apricots	Peaches	Strawberries
Oranges	Raspberries	Lemons

High

Apples	Currants	Plums
Bananas	Grapes	

VEGETABLES
Low

Asparagus	Cabbage Sprouts	Cauliflower
Brussels	Lettuce	Eggplant
Celery	Sauerkraut	Mushrooms
Green Peppers	Summer Squash	Spinach
Radishes	Beets	Swiss chard
String Beans	Pumpkin	Rutabaga
Tomatoes	Squash	Turnips
Onions	(Hubbard of	
Cucumbers	winter)	

Beet Greens	Broccoli	

High

Green peas	Lima beans	Parsnips
Corn	Potatoes	

D. STARCHES

Moderate

Tapioca
Bran

High

Bread	Crackers	Doughnuts
Rolls	Macaroni	Spaghetti
Noodles	Rice	Cereals:
		Corn flakes
		Shredded wheat
		Oatmeal

Note: "Low," "Moderate," and "High" refer to the relative amount of carbohydrates.

The QQF Theory

I presented my new QQF Theory for the etiology of obesity referring to quality, quantity, and frequency of the diet in June 1971 at the 120th Annual Convention of the American Medical Association, Atlantic City, New Jersey. In June 1972, it was again exhibited at the 121st A.M.A. Convention in San Francisco. It was first published in the Journal of the American Geriatrics Society in 1973. Over the years, it has been presented at several professional meetings and published in several professional journals. A complete listing may be found in the appendix. The QQF Theory considers not only the number of calories we eat but also the kind of food and the frequency of the meals. If you eat too many calories you may gain "weight," but whether that weight will be vital tissue or fat depends upon the QQF of your eating habits. *That you will lose "weight" by starving, there is no doubt*, but over half of the weight loss will be vital tissue essential for your health and well-being.

The number of carbohydrate calories you consume, in excess, is critical since they will cause a rise in blood sugar and subsequent storage of body fat. The protein and fat calories consumed will largely contribute to your lean body tissue and provide sustained energy sources. Once again, ingested fat will become body fat when elevated blood sugar levels promote insulin secretion by the pancreas. Therefore, the kind of food you eat is a much more critical factor than the amount of food in determining whether its destiny will be vital lean tissue or unwanted body fat.

The frequency of your meals is likewise important. If you eat at least three meals a day and avoid any feeling of fullness, you will not cause the liver glycogen storage to be exceeded and the excess blood sugar to be converted to body fat. Likewise, by having protein at each meal, you will ensure constant normal blood-sugar levels to the brain and nerves between meals and prevent the destruction of your vital lean tissues. Eating only one large meal per day will cause sarcopenic obesity, the accumulation of excess body fat with a simultaneous depletion of muscles and other vital lean tissues. Many obese people have sarcopenic obesity without even knowing it.

Toward A Healthier Life

All three—quality, quantity, and frequency of your food—are crucial. The time has come that we should all recognize this and stop limiting our thinking only to the number of calories we eat per day.

Even more important, the word *weight* must be replaced with the word *fat* in our vocabulary, since *it's excess body fat we want to lose*. Restricting sugars and refined starches to breakfast will automatically allow lipolysis, the movement of free fatty acids from stored body fat into the bloodstream, where they are carried by albumin to the muscles and other body cells to be used as aerobic energy.

Eating more unsaturated fats—in vegetable oils, and fish oils as well as saturated fat in butter in moderation—will increase the general metabolic rate and therefore increase the burning and loss of unwanted stored body fat.

When I say more unsaturated fat, specifically this means eating some fish five days a week and consuming 2 or 3 ounces of fish or vegetable oil daily. To some, this may seem excessive, but it will do the job. Dietary fats are an essential part of any successful diet for obesity. The secret which has yet to be recognized is *keeping dietary fats separated from sugars and refined starches*. Much more about this major breakthrough in the next chapter.

How do you determine which fats are largely saturated and which are largely unsaturated? The harder the fat on standing at room temperature, the more saturated it is. Lard and butter represent a higher degree of saturation, whereas vegetable and fish oils represent the unsaturated variety. A complete listing of the percentages of saturated fat vs. unsaturated fat is found in Table II in chapter 3.

Many people who want to get quick results in reducing may be unhappy enough with their condition to resort to crash-starvation methods. As we have seen, this only defeats their purpose, since more lean tissue (the tissue that burns fat as aerobic energy) is lost than is fat. Starvation is not an effective crash diet; rather it is pushing the "self-destruct button."

There is a "crash" diet that will work, and for those people who really want a crash program, the only safe and effective way is: *drink plenty of water, consume more vegetable oil, eat lean meat and fish, eat green vegetables, and have three small meals and two between-meal snacks a day.* For short periods, this may be an effective ready remedy. However, over the long haul, it is imperative that the diet system is designed to prevent boredom and assure adequate nutritional intake. This system has been presented in this chapter.

Restricting sugars, refined starches to breakfast; no sugars, fruits, or caffeine after breakfast; more essential oils; complete proteins at each meal—these are the tickets that will admit you to the theater of a better, happier, healthier life, one in which you will play your part more fully.

To Sum Up

1. You must eat three small meals and two between-meal protein-fat snacks a day.
2. Have some proteins at every meal. Choose egg, meat, shellfish, fish, fowl, or cheese—fish or meat, 3-5 ounces.
3. Limit your carbohydrates—eat up to 30 grams at breakfast and no more than 15-20 grams at the noon and evening meals.
4. Eat no carbohydrates between meals.
5. After breakfast, avoid all sugars, refined starches, and caffeine-containing foods.
6. Ingest 2 or 3 tablespoons of vegetable oil on a green salad at the noon and evening meals. Choose corn oil, safflower oil, canola oil, or olive oil.
7. Never be hungry or feel full when leaving the table following a meal.
8. There are no No-No's. All foods are allowed at breakfast.
9. Drink 6-8 8-oz. glasses of water a day.
10. Support vital tissue—lose excess fat pounds.

Chapter IX

Never After Breakfast

From the preceding chapter, you may have surmised that the diet I have recommended for you may have similarities to other diets. However, close scrutiny will reveal that it has a unique characteristic. This aspect I consider of great significance; in fact, it is the guarantee for your success in your battle against the bulge. The fact that all restaurants and hotels have served orange juice, doughnuts, coffee cakes and coffee at breakfast for hundreds of years is a universal testament to the body's need for sugars and starches at breakfast. One major reason why most all diets fail is there insistence for caloric restriction and their prohibition of certain food, i.e., sugars and refined starches and the high-calorie fats. Complete abstinence from sweets and refined starches is psychologically very difficult if not impossible. It will inevitably lead to rebellion in breaking the diet because your body has a real need for sugar at breakfast. After the overnight fast, your liver's glycogen (stored glucose) has been nearly depleted and therefore eating sugars and refined starches in moderation at breakfast will restore your liver's supply of glycogen.

Of course, the foundation of the diet propounded in this book: you are to *lose body fat*—not unspecified "weight."

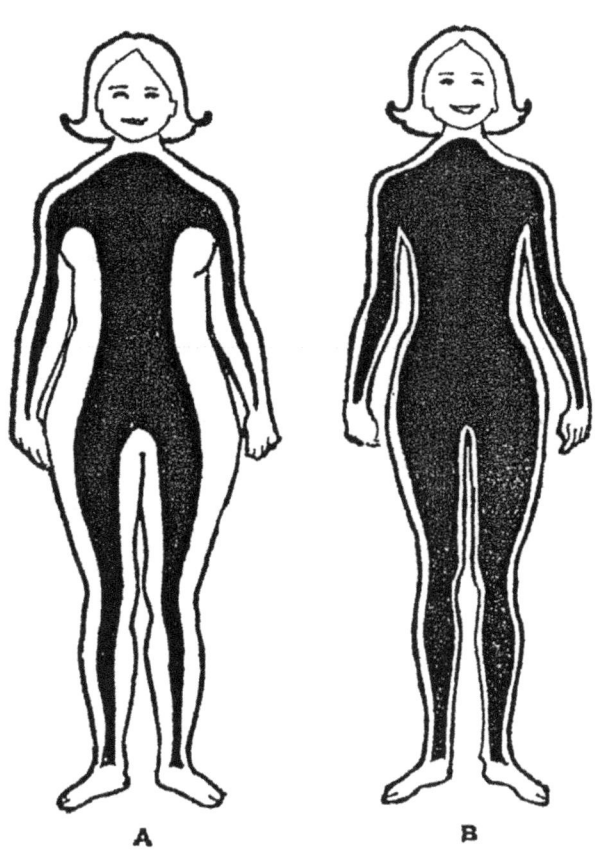

A   B

Almost everyone has been saying, "You've got to lose weight," "How many pounds have you lost?" A new slogan, which will be effective and get results, is *"Stop gaining*

135

more body fat." Many obese people are actually suffering from malnutrition and sarcopenic obesity. They are fat-laden but depleted of muscle and other vital tissues. By cutting calories, they lose "weight," but it may be predominantly from vital tissue.

To rid yourself of excess fat, the scientific way is to stop storing more fat by controlling your blood sugar and let your everyday activities and daily physical exercise gradually eliminate the unwanted fat excess. How is this done? We have seen, that fat in the form of free fatty acid is the major aerobic energy to the muscles and to other organs, such as the liver, kidney, and heart. Your body cells of these vital tissues burn fat as they sustain their existence and perform their functions.

See the illustration in Figure F. B has approximately twice the amount of vital tissue as A, but much less fat tissue. A appears to be much heavier than B, but in fact, they both may weigh the same. B's weight is primarily vital tissue, whereas A's is primarily fat. The simplest way to understand this is to look at a 130-pound young woman and a 130-pound young man. Both will weigh the same, but there should be no question about the difference in their appearance. The young lady has more body fat; the young man has more muscle. Assuming both A and B have the same metabolic rates, if A and B are sitting in a chair, *B may be burning up twice the amount of fat as A, since B has twice the number of muscle cells that burn fat as their primary aerobic energy.*

Now, no matter how much muscle and other vital tissues you have at this instance, if you stop producing any more fat, it should be obvious that in time, you will lose body fat in the everyday metabolic processes of your present vital tissues. Of course, by starving, you stop making fat and will lose some fat, but the catch is that you will also stop making and will lose vital tissues. In fact, the weight lost in starvation may be as much as two-thirds' vital tissue, and the dilemma is that the more vital tissues you lose, the less fat your body will burn as aerobic energy.

Getting back to the young man and woman. It has been said that girls are made of sugar and spice and everything nice. This appears to be partly true. Medical research has established that body fat is stored whenever the blood sugar rises sufficiently to induce insulin secretion. Sugars and sweets will raise blood sugar and contribute to the feminine contour.

Now, how do you stop storing more fat? The answer is—prevent your blood sugar from rising. If all sugars and starches become glucose, and when eaten in excess cause the blood sugar (glucose) to rise, and if caffeine causes the blood sugar to rise, does this mean that I should never eat sugars or caffeine? Not never, but NEVER AFTER BREAKFAST.

The time to eat doughnuts, coffee cake, fruits, jams, jellies, and yes, even pie, is at breakfast. In most of the best restaurants, desserts are served most always at breakfast. This has been a tradition in New England, in Mexico, in Greece, and in many other European countries.

One Portuguese lady told me there has been an old proverb for centuries in Portugal. "Oranges for breakfast are gold, for lunch are silver, and for supper are poison." When was the last time you drank orange juice for supper?

What's the medical explanation for eating sweets only at breakfast? Remember that the liver is the storage depot for sugar and holds only about 200-300 calories. At breakfast, the liver is nigh empty and eating sugars and refined starches serve to restore the liver's glycogen (stored glucose) supply. It requires a much longer time for the fats to reach a peak level in the bloodstream than it does for the sugar and refined starches. Therefore, the only safe time to eat the sweets, refined starches, and dietary fats together is at breakfast, when the blood fat level is at its lowest ebb. Later in the day, any rise in blood sugar will cause both blood sugars and fatty acids to be converted and stored as body fat.

This new slogan, "Never After Breakfast," is easy to remember, easy to enforce, and it works!

You can have sweets every day of your life at breakfast, but never after—and this will go very far in stopping your body from making and storing any more fat.

Again, caffeine must be limited to breakfast also. *Researchers at the Philadelphia General Hospital only recently discovered that caffeine will promote insulin secretion.* Caffeine is a central-nervous-system stimulant and will stimulate the adrenal glands to cause the liver to release its stored sugar into the bloodstream. At breakfast, the liver supply is at a very low ebb, so your morning cup of coffee can "wake you up" without causing the side reaction of spilling sugar into the bloodstream, where it can be converted into fat at the fat cell by insulin. And even if you do "succeed" in producing some fat at breakfast, it can be burned up as aerobic energy in the course of your daily activities.

Are fats fattening? Fats are fattening only in presence of alpha-glycerophosphate, a glucose metabolite present when the blood sugar rises and insulin is secreted by the pancreas. The saturated fats like butter and the visible fat on meat may be more fattening than the unsaturated oils and therefore should be limited in the diet. Therefore, cut the excess fat away from your steak.

What about water? Many hold fluids. If you are a water-holder, don't over-salt your foods. The exception here is in hot weather, when more salt may be necessary because it is readily lost by way of perspiration. Ironically, by drinking more water, less water is held by the body. You should drink 6-8 glasses of water per day.

At breakfast, you can eat anything in the grocery store. What about the "Ten Commandments" in chapter 8? The rules still apply and be sure to keep the daily 70-gram limit on carbohydrates. If your carbohydrate total at breakfast is over 30 grams, then cut down to a maximum of 15 grams at lunch and supper.

After breakfast, all fruits and food containing sugar, refined starches and caffeine are to vanish from your world. As far as you are concerned, they just don't exist. But you will always have something to look forward to—those "forbidden" sweets tomorrow morning. You may say, "That sounds easy, but can it be done?" It can be done by substituting. After breakfast, if you have a "sweet" tooth, substitute nuts. Make the habit of eating nuts when tempted to eat sweets.

After breakfast, for salt, a sodium-potassium mixture can be used; for butter, lean toward olive oil or canola oil; for coffee, use decaffeinated liquids.

What can you eat after breakfast? You may eat most vegetables at the lunch and evening meals as well as most nuts. In the vegetable group, watch out for *the big four— peas, corn, potatoes, and lima beans.* Also, closely watch the starches: bread, spaghetti, macaroni, and rice, etc. These starches will also promote a rise in blood sugar, causing you to store more body fat. Have some animal protein like egg yolk, meat, fish, fowl, or cheese at each meal, and with your lunch and supper, eat an oil-saturated green salad and other vegetables.

You should have two between-meal protein and fat-containing snacks a day, i.e., almonds or pork rinds. The rule is that between-meal snacks contain no carbohydrate and no caffeine.

Many people skip breakfast because they are not yet hungry. Farmers can teach us a lot about working up an appetite for breakfast. They go out and do their chores, then they are ready for their coffee, orange juice, hotcakes with syrup, a bowl of oatmeal, or bacon and eggs. What they are actually doing is waking the body, increasing the metabolic rate and the circulation and flow of digestive juice so that their bodies are ready to eat. Do your household chores, take a walk or jog around the block, exercise in your bedroom at least ten minutes before breakfast, and you will be surprised that you are not only able but eager to eat at the time when all foods are allowed.

What about calories? If you eat too many calories, you may gain "weight." But whether that weight is vital tissue, body fat, or water depends upon the what, how much of what, when and how often you eat, the QQF-quality, quantity, and frequency of your eating habits.

Sugar-containing calories are absolutely restricted to breakfast. Eat no carbohydrate-containing calories between meals. Eat more of the protein and essential-fat-containing calories and whole-grain starches in moderation at the noon and evening meals.

By gaining on the inside, vital tissues, you will be burning up more of your unwanted fat. By counting your grams of carbohydrate and never eating sugar, refined starches, or caffeine-containing foods after breakfast, you will not be gaining more body fat.

By gaining flesh, you will have the capacity to burn more body fat. *By gaining flesh, you can become trim, healthy, and attractive without sagging.* By never eating sugars after breakfast, you can remain trim and healthy. Is there some particular magic about certain fruits? Has grapefruit, for instance, a magic quality to cause weight reduction? No question that different fruits vary in their content of vitamins and minerals. This is why a variety in your fruit intake is urged; to assure a balance in your vitamin and mineral intake. But there's no weight-reduction magic in eating a particular fruit such as grapefruit. Switch around—have peaches, orange juice, bananas, berries, grapefruit, prunes, whatever—but only at breakfast. This principle of variety applies to all food, so, therefore, seek a wide variety in your protein and fat intake also. Your natural tastes should dictate to a large degree what particular food you select. But once more, in order to prevent yourself from producing fat, you must prevent your blood sugar from rising. Avoiding all fruits, sugars, refined starches, or caffeine-containing foods after breakfast is the way to accomplish this.

What happens if you do eat sugars and refined starches after breakfast? After breakfast, your liver may have become nearly filled with sugar (glycogen) from the carbohydrates you ate and from the proteins eaten which may have been converted to sugar. Ingestion of sugars and refined starches will cause the liver to spill over, the blood sugar to rise, and fat to be produced at every one of the countless fat cells in your body. And even worse, *the fat you consumed at breakfast circulates in the bloodstream for 8-10 hours.* It is there to act as substrata for rebuilding your vital tissue and as aerobic energy to the muscles, but if you raise the blood sugar by eating sweets, refined starches, and fruits or drinking caffeine, it will be transferred and stored as unwanted body fat. Mixing fat and sugar after breakfast—french-fried potatoes, peanut-butter-and-jelly sandwich, cake (contains sugar and shortening), and so on is a sure-fire way of making and storing body fat.

And as a double indemnity toward weight gain, when fat is produced from sugars, the body tends to hold water. Some Saturday afternoon, when you feel particularly indulgent, try eating a handful of candies and watch yourself puff up with water over the weekend. Better still, don't try it.

Keep the rule—no fruits, "sweets," refined starches or caffeine-containing foods are to be eaten after breakfast. Never after breakfast? Someone has said never say never. In obedience to this advice, you may eat ice cream and cake on birthdays and anniversaries. Some things could be more important than your figure. Also, during viral illnesses and colds, fruit juices may be very appealing after breakfast and are recommended. At that time, avoid eating fats to ensure that these two remain separated. *Keeping sugars and refined starches separated from dietary fats after breakfast is the key to your success in overcoming obesity without counting calories or eliminating any food from your diet.*

Breakfast means what it says, "breaking the fast." If you have fasted for 12-14 hours (the usual period from supper to breakfast), you may eat both sugars and fats together. After fasting this length of time the fat level in the bloodstream and the sugar level in the liver are both at very low ebbs. *Once you have broken the fast, then you must keep sugar and fat separated.* If the sugars are kept away from fat, then the fat you eat will be used as aerobic energy by the muscles and other vital tissues. But if ingested sugars and fats are allowed to combine after breakfast, the fat you eat will be stored as body fat.

I'll say it again—never eat sugars or refined starches or caffeine after breakfast. Keep this rule. If you break it, you can undo in one day what it may have taken you two weeks to accomplish. Two weeks of gradually burning up stored fat in the everyday metabolic processes could easily be undone in one day of "sweets" indulgence. The body has an awesome capacity to produce fat since every one of the billions of fat cells in your body is a miniature fat factory and fat is produced at the cell membrane of each of these cells whenever the blood sugar rises. On the other hand, it is very difficult to rid the body of the excess fat once it has been produced and stored. It has been estimated that if a strong man were to chop logs continuously for one hour, he would lose less than 3.2 ounces of fat.

Your carbohydrate counter (in the appendix) is divided into two sections: (1) carbohydrates that are never to be eaten after breakfast, and (2) carbohydrates that can be eaten at any meal but limited to a maximum number of grams.

The title of a song that appeared some years ago, "We Live in Two Different Worlds," expresses, in a nutshell, the dietary method I am advocating.

Your eating habits should be divided into two worlds: the world of breakfast and the world after breakfast. In your world of breakfast, anything goes, but in your world after breakfast sugars, refined starches, and caffeine-containing foods vanish, and you are to eat more of the fat-containing foods, more olive oil, avocados, nuts and butter, the protein-fat-containing foods—eggs, meat, fish, chicken, cheese; and more vegetables.

By keeping the sugars and fats separated in this manner and eating protein at every meal, you will accomplish the desired results of "gaining on the inside and losing on the outside."

These simple formulas:

Proteins + fats = flesh (muscle, kidney, blood, liver, glands, and other vital tissue)

Sugars + fats = body fat

—should be taught in kindergartens all over the world. Children should be taught to eat proteins and fats in order to rebuild and maintain their vital tissues in muscle, liver, and kidney, etc., but to eat foods containing sugar only at breakfast. If children were taught this at an early age, the continuing epidemic of obesity in our children would be prevented.

Chapter X
Physical Exercise

According to Dr. Jean Mayer, and colleagues at the Harvard School of Public Health, *one of the most important single causes of increased obesity in the United States today is the lack of physical exercise.*

When we recall that fat is the major source of aerobic energy to the muscles, it becomes clear why this statement may be true.

For years, it had been held that it really didn't make any difference how much we exercised, since the resultant increased appetite would only produce an augmented caloric intake that would nullify any weight loss resulting from physical exertion. This was before the knowledge became known, that in reality *there are two major energy systems in the body: the nervous system, requiring sugar (glucose), and the muscles and majority of other lean body cells, requiring fat (free fatty acid) for aerobic energy. Sugar (glucose) is stored in the muscles as glycogen to be used as a secondary energy.*

We have all observed how some children eat anything they want but may not become obese. Yes, they do turn the sugars and starches into fat, but may burn it up in that very,

very active phase of their life. Children who have been deprived of essential dietary fats, because they are high in calories will be *hungry* and eat sugars and starches in excess resulting in obesity. Several of my patients have told me that they had been always hungry until they started including the essential fats in butter, olive oil, canola oil, and the fat in meat and fish in their diet. Your body has a very real need for these essential fats and including them in your diet appeases your appetite.

The thin silhouette cast by most distance runners and professional dancers can be attributed to the same principle. Physical exercise is a sure way of losing body fat.

The secret of successful exercising is daily repetition, and therefore short intervals repeated without fail daily are much to be desired over sporadic strenuous exercise. Exercises requiring only ten minutes a day designed to add strength and suppleness to the muscles of the entire body are listed as follows:

1. Warm-Ups
   a. Run in place for one minute.
   b. Starting Position: Stand with arms at sides.
      Action: Jump to a straddle stand, clap hands overhead, count 1 return 2.
2. Hip Suppling
   a. Starting Position: straddle stand (heels wide apart), arms at sides, bend forward, left hand to left foot, right hand to right foot count 1, stay there, emphasize this movement count 2, again on 3, and straighten on count 4.

b. Starting Position: Stand on left knee, right leg forward, the heel on the floor, arms at side.

Action: Reach forward, touch right toes with hands 1, stay there and emphasize this movement on 2, again on 3, return to starting position count 4 (repeat 16 counts with left leg forward).

3. Shoulder Suppling

a. Starting Position: Stand with arms upward (arms straight, thumbs point to the rear, palms toward each other.

Action: From this position, jerk arms backward vigorously count 1, again 2, again 3, to a starting position on 4.

b. Starting Position: Straddle stand, left hand on hip, right arm hanging to the side, hand closed to a loose fist.

Action: Swing right arm forward upward to the ceiling, continue this making a circle, now continue with 7 more circles. Repeat with the opposite arm.

4. Lateral Trunk

a. Starting Position: Straddle stand, arms upward, hands one foot apart.

Action: Bend trunk directly to the left side, count 1, straighten up on count 2, repeat 1-2, right side 3-4 (note: hands to remain one foot apart even when bending trunk).

b. Starting Position: Stand on left knee, right leg sideward, arms overhead, hands on foot apart.

Action: Bend trunk directly to side, repeat 16 times right and 16 times left.

5. General Trunk

   a. Starting Position: Straddle stand, arms sideward, reach for walls. Action: move the left hand to right foot count 1, return to starting position count 2, repeat to opposite side 3 and 4.

   b. Starting Position: Straddle stand, trunk bent forward, left fist on the floor between feet, right fist to the ceiling.
   Action: Change arm positions, the right arm comes down, left goes up (trunk twisting). Repeat for 10 counts.

6. Posterior Trunk

   a. Starting Position: Lying on the floor (face down) arms sideward, palms on the floor.
   Action: Raise arms, head, chest, feet, hold count 1-2-3, return 4 (swan-dive position).

   b. Starting Position: Front lying position on the floor, hand on hand, under forehead (forehead resting on top hand).
   Action: From this position, raise both legs (straight) upward, hold position count 1-2-3, lower to the floor, count 4.

7. Abdominal

   a. Starting Position: Lying flat on the back, arms crossed on chest, feet together.
   Action: Raise head, shoulders and back to 45 degrees, count 1-2-3, return to lying position

count 4 (hold feet or hook toes under stationary object).

b.　Starting Position: From lying position flat on the back, knees bent and hands behind head (it will be necessary for someone to hold feet or root toes under stationary object.

Action: Raise trunk upward to sitting position count 1, return to a lying position, count 2 slowly.

8.　Arm Strengthening

a.　Starting Position: On hands and knees (a distance of about 2 feet between hands and knees) (women only).

Action: Bend arms and raise straight, the left leg to the ceiling. Keep elbows off floor count 1, return count 2, repeat arms bend. Raise opposite leg count 3, return 4.

b.　Starting Position: Front support lying (pushup position) (men only).

Action: Bend arms, lower body until one inch off the floor. Count 1, straighten arms, count 2, repeat for 10 counts, rest for 10 counts. Repeat.

9.　Leg Strengthening

a.　Starting Position: Straight stand, hands behind head.

Action: Bend knees, slowly count 1-2-3-4, straighten knees slowly 5-6-7-8, and repeat.

b.　Starting Position: Straddle stand, arms sideward or hold table or chair for balance.

Action: Bend left knee (lowering seat to left heel), count 1-2-3, straighten knee 4. Repeat opposite 5-6-7-8.

10. Head (Neck)
   a. Starting Position: Seated on the floor, hands on the upper leg (thigh).

   Action: Turn head as far left as possible on count 1, right on count 2. Look upward to ceiling count 3, lower head forward count 4.

   b. Starting Position: Lying position flat on the back, arms sideward and palms on the floor, as a. from this position.

11. Relaxing
   a. Starting Position: Lying flat on the back, arms overhead, with palms to the ceiling.

   Action: Stretch (make yourself as tall as possible) moving hands out overhead, feet in the opposite direction. Make yourself tall count 1, relax 2.

Give one minute to each exercise.

Courtesy of Professor W. C. Eberhard, former Director Physical Education, St. Louis University. St. Louis, Missouri.

Aside from causing a reduction in body fat, exercise is very beneficial for your health. *It increases the general efficiency of the body's working parts by a general increase in circulation and respiration. Hence, nutrients carried in the bloodstream and oxygen inhaled from the air are supplied in greater quantity to all body cells dependent for their survival.* And daily exercise is essential to derive the greatest benefit for tissue building from the food you eat.

Striking proof of the necessity of exercising for the assimilation of foodstuffs is vividly demonstrated whenever we cast a limb that had been fractured. When the cast is removed from an arm, for instance, after a period of six to eight weeks, the muscles will be withered and the joints will have become stiffened. Only through exercise and proper nutrition will the muscles and joints return to their normal status. A leg that is cast may sometimes appear larger after the cast is removed since it has "filled" with water, but the muscle will be atrophied, demonstrated by weakness and inability to use it normally. *Inactivity, then, causes wasting of muscles even though the diet may be adequate.*

It has been established that daily exercise tends to diminish the chances of having heart disease, and in addition, our bodies become conditioned to a greater degree of efficiency, giving us more zest and vitality for living and the enjoyment of recreation in general.

The only truly beneficial form of exercise is active exercise—that kind in which the person is using his own muscles. Passive exercise—that is performed upon us either by massage or machine—may have benefits with regard to some increase in circulation but is of practically no value in causing a reduction of body fat. We lose little fat by way of apparatuses but must earn our daily fat loss by the sweat of our brow.

The dilemma in which the overweight person finds himself is that he is told to count calories and start running. This is something like strapping a fifty-pound weight on the shoulders of a mile trackman and training him by depriving him of nutritious foods.

It is essential that we realize that many overweight people are that skinny miler carrying fifty and more pounds of excess fat tissue. They must have the muscle tissues restored and maintained before they can engage in exercise, which will produce the desired loss of body fat.

Over-exercising the sarcopenic obese is a hazardous process. Because of depleted vital tissues and excessive fat loads, very strenuous exercise can produce collapse and even precipitate a heart attack.

My advice is to pick up your step in walking, walk more often, and for longer distances. Running, jogging, or the daily systematic total body exercises given in this chapter are recommended, but should be discontinued at any noticeable shortness of breath. In the beginning, do only the "a" series of exercises and as your strength and endurance gain, gradually take on the "b" series.

A major value of daily exercise is that it will tone your muscles, and thus tend to change your flab and sag to trim. The general overall efficiency of the body physiology will be increased and the condition generally sought for, fitness, will be more readily achieved.

We have come to understand that our body's energy system can be compared to char in an auto, our "gasoline" being body fat and our "electricity" being blood sugar (glucose). You burn more gas by accelerating your engine. Exercise will accelerate the action of your muscles and increase the metabolism causing more fat "gasoline" to be burned as energy. And it has been experimentally shown that short exercise periods will increase the general metabolic rate for hours following the exercise period. This is decidedly beneficial in promoting small but certain losses of body fat.

For years' glucose was considered to be the sole energy of the body. It is now established that glucose stored in the muscles as glycogen is a secondary energy used during exercises where the oxygen supply is insufficient such as weight lifting and sprinting. For better fitness, anaerobic exercise may serve as a valuable addition to an aerobic exercise regimen. Of course, before engaging in any physical exercise regimen, a check-up with your physician is advised.

Fat, to be sure, is a very efficient source of energy, and any noticeable loss of dimensions through exercise will take its time appearing, but be assured that *whenever you move a muscle, some fat is being "burned" in the process.*

Most overweight people are tense and tired. Exercise is a ready answer to relieve fatigue and ease tensions. It may seem paradoxical, but by burning energy, new energy can be yours. You will stay on top by getting fit. Better appearance, greater happiness, less proneness to illness can all be yours by developing the daily exercise habit.

A physical checkup from your doctor should precede any active exercise program.

Many people do not eat and do not want breakfast. This is your most important meal. You will want breakfast if you play this little game—tell yourself the ticket for starting your day is your exercise routine. Do it or you don't go out of your bedroom. After your exercises, take a hot shower and rinse off in an invigorating cold shower, summer and winter, every day. You will soon find how enjoyable breakfast is and what it does for you. And remember, breakfast is where you can eat any food you like. There are no "no-nos" at breakfast.

Daily exercise will give you more flexibility and increased ability in your favorite sport, and if you remember that the calories burned up in exercise are largely from your body fat stores, you may find this a real incentive to work harder and play harder.

In order to work and play harder, you've got to have energy. It has been proven that caloric restrictions will lower the metabolism and will cause you to fatigue easily and have less energy. Your diet supplies all the energy necessary and then some for efficient work and play activity. Thus, there are no hunger pangs. Therefore, with ample energy and absence of hunger, there will be little reason for you to break away from your way of eating as outlined in Chapter 8.

In Table IV are listed a relative scale of calories representing the amount of free fatty acids (fat) mobilized from the fat cells and oxidized by the muscles as energy during sports and ordinary activities.

Table IV

CALORIC COST OF
DAILY LIVING ACTIVITIES
AND SPORTS
(For Periods of Motion Only)
Calories per Minute per sq. Meter of Body Surface

Normal activity		Sport	
Sitting, normal	0.70	Football	5.04
Sitting, reading	0.70	Basketball	4.31
Sitting, eating	0.80	Bowling	4.06
Sitting, playing cards	0.83	Swimming	6.06
Resting in bed	0.68	Golfing	2.76
Standing, normal	0.81	Tennis	3.50
Standing, light activity	1.41	Squash	5.00
Personal toilet	1.09	Table Tennis	2.00
Shower	1.84	Badminton	1.91
Dressing	1.84	Towing	4.00
Making beds	2.64	Sailing	1.30
Shining shoes	2.11	Snooker pool	1.50
Mopping floors	2.67	Dancing	2.00
Walking indoors	1.68	Riding	1.50
Walking outdoors	3.07	Boxing, sparring	5.00
Walking upstairs	10.00		

Walking downstairs	3.80
Kneeling	0.68
Squatting	1.12
Washing	1.42

Chapter XI

Self-Hypnosis For A New Body Image

We have faced facts: one of the biggest obstacles to overcoming obesity is the misapplied Caloric Theory—and along with it, a host of misguided ideas about "weight loss." You know that attempting to rid yourself of excess body fat by calorie-cutting will never get the job done. Indeed, it may deplete your lean vital tissues and ultimately generate more body fat. You must "feed the lean but starve the fat." It's the way to become—and *remain*—trim, healthy and attractive.

Understanding these facts is crucial to overcoming obesity. Yet, there is still one more stumbling block that deserves considerable attention.

Just Imagine!

When people struggle with obesity, it is often because they rely almost solely upon will power. However, you possess a faculty that is far more powerful than will: your imagination. Whenever will and imagination are in conflict, imagination *will* win out.

The sure-fire way to accomplish any fear is to visualize yourself succeeding before actually starting. In fact, this is how many athletes prime themselves for competition, using visualization to get into "the zone." Whereas will power is a faculty of your conscious mind, imagination dwells within your subconscious mind where more of your personal power resides. Using the will exclusively is tiring. Only the strongest can rely on it alone, stay the course and achieve their goals. Those with weaker wills—the majority of us—can accomplish more by taking advantage of the great power of our imaginations.

To understand imagination's dominance of the will, do this brief experiment: try not to think of an elephant. No doubt, an elephant has already popped into your mind. In fact, the more you try not to think of the elephant, the more vivid it becomes, right?

Hypnosis is a very practical and effective way of tapping the power of your imagination. However, before we explore hypnosis, I have another thought-experiment for you: Consider what you would look like without any skin or body fat. Looking at yourself, what would you see? Take a few moments and really put forth your best effort in providing an answer. We'll return to the question a bit later in this chapter.

The Truth About Trance

Only within the past few decades has hypnosis emerged from the cloak of mysticism under which it has been deemed only something to be feared or shunned. Now, its true nature and value are being appreciated and utilized. In fact, the medical, dental and psychological professions all have endorsed the use of hypnosis as a therapeutic modality to alleviate and correct numerous maladies and conditions. Still, there are many misconceptions in both the lay and professional communities which should be addressed.

First, without cooperation and willingness on the part of the subject, a hypnotist cannot hypnotize anyone. Rather, the hypnotist acts as a guide, teaching the subject how to cross over from the normal waking state into the condition of mind known as *trance*. The subconscious mind can be given suggestions so one can accomplish feats that, while in the waking state, seem impossible. For, though having the strength of a giant, the subconscious mind has the will of a small child. If the suggestions given to it during trance are acceptable, your subconscious mind can transform them into reality. Crucially, your subconscious mind will reject those suggestions that are repugnant to you or violate your moral values.

There are two prerequisites for entering the trance state. First, you consent to be hypnotized. If you do not want it to happen, hypnosis will not occur. Second, you must be free of fear and mistrust of the process or the hypnotist. In choosing a physician or a hypnotist, select one who is both qualified and trustworthy. It would be unwise to allow just anyone to bring you into a trance. And despite the numerous performers who purport to hypnotize audience members for entertainment purposes, hypnosis is not a parlor trick to be used for amusement. It is a serious and very useful therapeutic tool.

When you are in trance, though you may appear to be unconscious, you will be in control of all of your faculties except for what may be termed your "critical faculty." You will be able to see, hear, smell, taste, feel and speak. You will have complete awareness of your surroundings, but your critical faculty will be bypassed. That is, if a pleasing and acceptable, emotionally and morally reasonable suggestion is given to you, you will accept it and act upon it, even though in your normal, waking state you might consider it an impossibility. For example, while you are in trance, an anesthetic effect might be suggested for your hand, and you would be completely impervious to pain at that site. A needle could pierce the skin of your hand without your experiencing any discomfort whatsoever. Or, you might be "taken back" to an early age, say five years old, and you would be able to see with your mind's eye, in very accurate detail, everything that occurred at the particular instance you were directed to "relive."

Of course, your attitudes and beliefs about yourself can be dramatically changed by hypnosis, and this has profound implications for the treatment of obesity.

You Are What You Think

Though more than 40 years in family and obesity practice, I have learned that many who have problems with obesity have a fat self-image. They have always seen themselves as *being* fat, and they think they will stay that way. While they may consciously seek to "lose weight," their subconscious minds have been programmed to fulfill the image of being and remaining fat. Positive change seems impossible. Meanwhile, they keep getting the time-worn advice, "Stop eating so much! Cut calories! It's the *only way*!" Thus are they doubly doomed, for not only are they set up for failure by their subconscious mindset but by what has proven to be ineffective: cutting calories to "lose weight." Doubtless, that obsolete notion has got to go before any progress can be made, even with hypnosis. But illuminated by the facts about obesity, the marvelous instrument of hypnosis can change a fat self-image into one that is trim, healthy and attractive, and help make that new self-image into a permanent reality.

Beyond having a distorted body image, many fat people may be punishing themselves—and others—due to unresolved guilt or feelings of hostility. Their causes may be repressed from memory and may have occurred as far back as early childhood. Such feelings are submerged in the depths of the subconscious mind like a tetherball tied at the bottom of a dark lake. Under hypnosis, the mighty subconscious can cut the cord, allowing the causative more impersonally, thus weakening its destructive effect. Until this conscious awareness is achieved, however, the incident will continue to devastate, no matter how long ago the original incident occurred.

To impress upon you the power of hypnosis, let me briefly tell you of another patient. Although her story is not directly related to our concern with obesity, its searing lessons are.

"Heather" was a 25-year-old woman who sought my services because her life had become nearly intolerable. She was contemplating suicide. Her home was filled with Tupperware and almost every other object offered by salespeople who had come to her door. At her job, she stayed late nearly every evening, typing the work readily heaped upon her by the other secretaries. After all, she always seemed so willing to help. Thus, once word got around that Heather never refused a proposition, her male acquaintances took advantage of her.

Under hypnosis, Heather was taken back in time to "relive" the incident that was responsible for all of this self-destructive behavior. In a trance, she described what she saw in her mind's eye: herself as a little girl in the kitchen, banging together pots and pans, making a terrific noise. Her mother stormed in and snarled, "Are you going to stop making that noise?"

As any child at that age might respond, she declared, "No!"

Her mother grabbed her and yanked her up to her face. She screamed, "Don't you ever say no to me or anyone else."

This statement was imprinted on Heather's subconscious mind and was to render its devastating effects upon her until the day it was finally brought to her conscious awareness through hypnosis. Its voltage thus dissipated by awareness of why she could never refuse any request, her life changed completely. She became quite able to say "no" whenever she deemed it the proper response. Such a wonderful recovery was made possible by hypnosis. Indeed, there may be no other way that it could have occurred.

Hypnosis may be similarly effective for those who continue to eat compulsively because of repressed events. Some may harbor deep feelings of resentment from past hurts, traumas which may also be repressed. Such people may use their obesity as a way of striking back—ironically, by hurting themselves and possibly others who may have had nothing to do with the original harm. Hypnosis may give such people insight, then, and finally allow them to become the trim, healthy and attractive people they have always wanted to be.

Why hypnosis? *Hypnosis is the one known modality wherein direct contact can be made with the subconscious mind—the storehouse for all of life's past experiences and the powerhouse where the "impossible" becomes possible.*

What Do You See?

Since the main job of a hypnotist is actually to guide you into the stare of trance, you can learn how to enter the trance state by self-hypnosis. The rest of this chapter explains how to do so and further your achievement of a trim and healthy body.

But first, let us finish our thought-experiment. The question was if you could see yourself without any skin or body fat, what would you see? The answer: you would see your heart, lungs, muscles, liver, spleen, kidneys, glands, intestines, and blood vessels . . . Was that your answer? I have asked many of my patients this same question, and most of them have difficulty answering it. We easily forget the magnificent body machinery operating just under the skin. After all, when you look at someone, how often do you "see" that person's heart or lungs or muscles? But this is what you have to learn to do now with respect to your own body: *see in your mind's eye all the working parts of your own body and realize that to become trim and healthy, you must eat in such a way as to nourish those working parts*

163

while simultaneously starving the fat on your body. This is the essence of understanding and overcoming the obesity problem. Forget about "cutting calories to lose weight," you now know, the very notion of "losing weight' is off the mark. Think about gaining weight—*on the inside*—nourishing your inner vital lean tissues in muscles, liver, kidney, etc., while losing your outer coat of body fat.

Self-Hypnosis: A Guide

Find a room where you can be alone and undisturbed. Lie down and get comfortable. Close your eyes and roll them back as though you were trying to look into the top of your head. Take a very deep breath and let it out slowly. Take another deep breath and pay attention to the silent "inner voice" that only you can hear. With your silent inner voice, give yourself the following suggestions. Let the suggestions come from your conscious mind talking to the inner you. That is, address your subconscious mind in the second person, as "you" instead of "I." In this way, you will be giving suggestions directly to your subconscious mind and by bypassing the critical faculty of your conscious mind, you will produce the desired result.

Relaxed now and breathing slowly and deeply, "speak" to your inner subconscious mind, with your silent voice:

Close your eyes, now focus your entire attention on your eyelid muscles. These muscles are very tiny and very easy to control. Now let those tiny eyelid muscles go loose and limp, perfectly relaxed. Relax them perfectly and completely. Just as you can make a muscle so tight that it won't work, you can also make a muscle so loose that it won't work. So, let those tiny muscles in your eyelid go loose and limp, and perfectly relaxed. Relax them to the point where they will not work, they will not open. And when you're sure—and be sure in your own mind—convince yourself so that you know that those tiny eyelid muscles are so loose and so limp and so relaxed that they simply will not work—they will not open. When you are certain of this, test them and see that they will not work—they will not open.

You will find that your eyes will not open, no matter how hard you try, and you will know that you have entered the hypnotic trance.

Continue to relax your whole body. With your silent voice, say,

Send that relaxation you have in your eyelids all throughout your body. Feel it spread all the way down to the tips of your toes and the ends of your fingers, and notice how good that feels.

You'll be very pleasantly surprised by just how good you will feel.

Now, you can take yourself deeper into the hypnotic trance. Say with your inner voice,

Raise your right arm toward the ceiling and notice it getting stiffer and stiffer, stiffer and stiffer. Now it's as stiff as a board and you can't bend it. The more you try to bend it, the stiffer it will be.

Try to bend your arm. You will find that it will not bend, despite your best effort. Having confirmed that you are indeed in a trance state, you can relax your arm by saying with your inner voice,

The muscles in your right arm are now relaxing, slowly lower your right arm and let it rest in your lap, loose and limp like a wet dishrag.

You are now ready to give your subconscious mind suggestions that will bring to fruition the promise of becoming trim, healthy and attractive. Continue with your inner voice directed to your subconscious mind,

You now realize that counting calories to lose weight can never get the job done for you. What you really want is to become trim, healthy, and attractive and stay that way. So, see the image of that trim, healthy and attractive person you've always wanted to be in your mind's eye right now and keep that image, believing it will become a reality.

With practice, you will be able to "see" your new body image. Now say with your inner voice,

Imagine yourself gradually becoming that trim, healthy and attractive person you've always wanted to be. Keeping that image in your mind's eye and following the QQF Lifetime Way of Eating, and notice—as the days and weeks go by—how much happier and more confident you become as you see the excess fat disappearing from your body. Becoming trim, healthy and attractive is not only a function of eating but of attitude. Recognize that you have made the choice to become and that remain trim, healthy and attractive, and take pride in realizing you are now in control of your new eating habits. Avoid measuring success in terms of how much weight you lose each week, but allow your appearance, better health, new values towards food and changed eating patterns to help you stay with The QQF Way. What you eat, how much of what you eat, when and how often you eat will make your new body image become a reality.

All of the productive suggestions having been made, it is now time to "wake yourself up." So continue with your inner voice,

Now, as you look forward to the new figure and better health you know you are going to have, at the count of three you will be alert, clear-headed and refreshed-and feeling just fine. With your inner voice count: 1... 2... becoming alert... and 3. Open your eyes. Feeling just fine.

At this suggestion, you will indeed emerge from the trance, alert, clear-headed and refreshed.

Having the means to hypnotize yourself, you have an even stronger beginning towards becoming—and remaining—trim, healthy and attractive, making your dream a reality. Memorize the above suggestions and direct them to your subconscious mind, but don't worry if you can't remember them word for word. What's important is to impress their meaning upon your subconscious mind. And you needn't limit yourself to these suggestions. You may well want to add suggestions of your own. The only rule for making suggestions is this: they must be expressed in positive terms. Your subconscious mind will gloss right over the negative. For example, if your suggestion is, "Don't eat sugars and refined starches after breakfast," your subconscious mind will ignore the "don't" and hear only the message, "Eat sugars and refined starches after breakfast." To suggest this in the positive is to say something like, "Eat sugars and starches only at breakfast" or "Avoid sugars and starches after breakfast."

You should practice self-hypnosis someplace where you will not be disturbed. You may even want to unplug or turn off your phone during the time you will be hypnotized. However, if this is not practical or desirable if the phone should ring or an emergency occurs while you are in trance, you can wake yourself rapidly by saying with your silent voice, "1, 2, 3, wake up," and you will do so at once, fully alert.

Let It Happen

The goal for getting the best results with self-hypnosis is to "just let it happen." The more you practice, the more easily you will be able to hypnotize yourself, the "deeper" you will be able to go and the more potent and effective the results will be. You will be well on your way to becoming—and remaining—that trim, healthy and attractive person you visualize each time you hypnotize yourself.

As suggested, hypnosis can be used for many purposes beyond improving your physical appearance and health. It can improve your sports skills, your memory and ability to perform almost any endeavor. It can bolster your self-confidence, enable you to relax, free yourself of tensions, anxieties, fears, and help you fall asleep effortlessly. Hypnosis can eliminate or lessen pain or headaches, control asthma, help you overcome bad habits such as smoking or excessive drinking.

You may wonder how such a wonderful modality could have thus far passed you by. You needn't wonder. Just help yourself.

Please check with your family physician regarding the advisability of your using self-hypnosis as a therapeutic modality.

Chapter XII

Diseases Associated With Obesity

It is a cliché that the fat man is a jolly man. Any obese person knows down deep that this is untrue. Usually, when looking in the mirror, he or she is not admiring his or her features but is doing so for another reason—to shave, apply makeup, pluck an eyebrow, or whatever. In actuality, few obese people see their reflection. They avoid it because they do not like what they would see. Emotional problems riddle their lives. They feel inferior, unwanted, and rejected and a great many have hostile feelings. Little wonder—unable to cross their legs, forced to buy special clothing, feeling guilty whenever they put a bite of food in their mouths. If the emotional problems were the only problems, obesity would be a tragedy, but added to this are many physical problems that contribute to a whole array of disease and morbidity states (Figure G).

Obesity is the number-one health problem in the United States today.

Statistics have conclusively revealed that excess body fat will shorten the life span—heart disease being the major problem.

Let's remember that obesity is defined as that condition wherein *a person has accumulated excess body fat. The excess fat must be nourished by blood capillaries that add miles of vessels through which the blood must be pumped.* This puts a constant strain on the heart muscle and after several years may result in an enlarged heart. The added mileage of blood vessels also may force a compensatory increase in force, which will result in high blood pressure. Almost invariably, the patients I have successfully treated for obesity have shown a drop in their blood pressure.

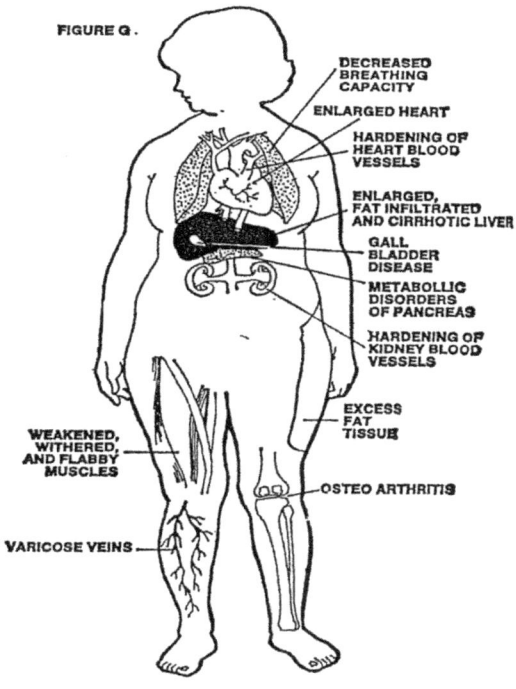

FIGURE G.

DECREASED BREATHING CAPACITY

ENLARGED HEART

HARDENING OF HEART BLOOD VESSELS

ENLARGED, FAT INFILTRATED AND CIRRHOTIC LIVER

GALL BLADDER DISEASE

METABOLLIC DISORDERS OF PANCREAS

HARDENING OF KIDNEY BLOOD VESSELS

EXCESS FAT TISSUE

OSTEO ARTHRITIS

WEAKENED, WITHERED, AND FLABBY MUSCLES

VARICOSE VEINS

DISEASE CONDITION ASSOCIATED WITH OBESITY

Heart Conditions

A major vital concern to us all at this time is coronary arteriosclerosis, the thickening and hardening of the inner lining of the heart vessels—a condition that may lead to a "heart attack." A heart attack is that condition where a major heart artery has been occluded and hence the portion of the heart muscle nourished by this vessel will die. The severe pain associated with this can cause shock and death.

A tremendous amount of research has been done in seeking the answer for the cause of coronary arteriosclerosis and myocardial infarction, or heart attack. There has been statistical evidence that elevated serum cholesterol levels may be a predisposing factor, and hence excessive amounts of cholesterol-containing foods have been restricted in patients with heart disease. *The ingestion of excessive amounts of saturated fats may promote a rise in serum cholesterol, whereas the unsaturated oils will promote a decrease in serum cholesterol levels—thus my previous recommendation to eat fat in the ratio of two unsaturated to one saturated.*

It has been recently shown that *people who eat little fat and excessive amounts of sugars will have elevated levels of serum triglyceride and low-density lipoprotein. These are more indicative of a risk for coronary heart disease than is elevated total cholesterol.*

And it is a well-known fact that concentrated sugars injected into an artery will have a very definite sclerosing effect. Researchers have isolated an infective organism in the artery walls that may cause damage to the internal lining of the vessel wall, development of plaques, and eventual rupture, and blockage of the artery. *This particular organism has an affinity for sugar,* and therefore, aside from promoting obesity, sugar in excess may be a major predisposing agent that may lead to a heart attack.

The metabolic syndrome, defined as a cluster of conditions including obesity, high blood pressure, elevated serum triglyceride, and LDL cholesterol and elevated serum glucose levels, commonly precedes the development of chronic heart disease and diabetes and poses a definite risk for myocardial infarction, heart attack. Recent research has suggested that a low glycemic, moderate protein and fat diet may reverse the metabolic syndrome.

Diabetes

In general, there are two types of diabetic patients: the juvenile and the mature onset. Most of the true juvenile diabetics are thin and require insulin for their management. Over 80 percent of diabetics are obese and have been classified as mature onset or Type II variety, usually occurring in the early forties. But now, the great majority of obese diabetic children have Type II diabetes and the great majority of obese diabetic patients have excess serum-insulin levels. And since insulin is necessary for body fat production, the correlation between obesity and Type II diabetes can be readily recognized.

Diabetes is a most serious disease, since most diabetics may have some degree of arteriosclerosis, which if severe can predispose to a heart attack. Blindness or loss of toes, a foot, or even a leg can occur in severe cases.

The primary requisite in the treatment and prevention of diabetes is the limiting of sugars and refined starches in the diet.

Other Common Problems

Excessive fat in the mesentery of the intestines will crowd the diaphragm upward and therefore cause a serious limitation of the lungs' expanding capability, making it difficult for the obese person to inhale vital oxygen and exhale waste in the form of carbon dioxide. Yet, the "message" regarding the treatment of obesity has been: "eat less and start running." I have told many patients that suppose I invent a contraption, a canvas sack containing thirty pounds of sand; strap it on their back, lock it in place, and then tell them to eat less and start running. What do you think would happen to them?

Many unfortunate obese patients may have, not thirty pounds, but as many as one hundred pounds of body fat weighing them down and crowding their lungs. Moreover, their muscles may be flabby and withered as the result of prolonged abstinence from protein and certain essential fats in the diet.

The weight of the excess body fat can cause continual trauma to the joints of the body, particularly in the feet, knees, and hips, and may result in painful and crippling arthritis.

Redundant fat may interfere with the venous return of the blood from the legs and result in unsightly varicose veins.

Fatty liver and cirrhosis of the liver are other common problems in the obese. Attempts to reduce by extreme caloric restriction will result in depletion of the liver vital cells, fatty infiltration in the liver, and eventually may scar into a cirrhotic liver.

Gallbladder disease is very often noted in the female or male who is fat and forty.

Their heavy coat of fat makes it very difficult for obese people to keep cool in the summer.

Obstetrical and surgical risks, as well as postoperative morbidity, are increased substantially because of excessive adiposity, the medical term for body fat.

Relation to Cancer

As for the most dreaded of all diseases, cancer, statistics have long linked the presence of certain cancers with obesity, but now direct laboratory evidence has demonstrated that an organism classified as mycobacterium seems to have an affinity for sugar and may be a causal agent of cancer.

Doctors Virginia Livingston and Eleanor Jackson pioneered the research that led to the discovery of this microbe, and the culmination of their twenty years' work appeared in the September 1965 issue of the *Journal of the American Medical Women Association,* with photographs of the microbe they had isolated in many human cancers. This microbe metamorphoses into various forms, including viruses, bacteria, and yeast-like forms, which is why, according to the investigators, it had never before been identified. Since the mycobacterium microbe, called

Mycobacterium tumefaciens, may feed on sugar, these doctors advocate the restriction of carbohydrates, particularly sugars and refined starches, in patients being treated for cancer. The use of the Tuberculosis BCG vaccine to cause remission in melanoma, leukemia, and cancer of the bladder, tends to substantiate the claims of Doctors Livingston and Jackson, since the tuberculosis microbe is from the same genus, *Mycobacterium,* as the microbe they have suggested is a cause for cancer.

Low Blood Sugar

Complaints from obese patients include fatigue, sweating, rapid heartbeat, headache, dizziness, muscle pains, blurred vision, numbness, anxiety, depression, insomnia, irritability, unsocial or antisocial behavior, and restlessness. A possible cause of these symptoms could be relatively low blood sugar, which ironically, can be brought about by eating sugar and refined starches and drinking sugar and caffeine-containing liquids. The blood sugar may rise sharply causing insulin secretion, then drops to a low level, having been converted into fat, and it is then that these symptoms are experienced by the patient. For parents (particularly the obese) diagnosed as having hyperinsulinism with subsequent hypoglycemia (low blood sugar), sugar and caffeine are prohibited in the diet. In addition, there has been recent evidence to substantiate the supposition that the symptoms of schizophrenia may be in part related to recurrent hypoglycemia.

Malnutrition and Obesity

It would be well to recognize that there are two classifications of obese patients, the over-nourished obese and the undernourished obese. Obesity in either form is undesirable. The latter has been classified as having sarcopenic obesity. People with sarcopenic obesity have excess body fat with concurrent depleted, withered, and flabby musculature. They are prone to arthritis, anemia and have poor resistance to infections. Suffering from malnutrition, they must eat more proteins and certain fats to regain and maintain lost vital tissue but less of the carbohydrates to prevent adding to their fat load. The proper way to do this, I believe, has been presented in previous chapters.

The problem of obesity in our country and indeed many parts of the world has reached a critical point, and a solution to the problem is necessary to improve the health of the people of today and ensure the health of generations to come. The principles in this book may provide such a solution.

To Sum Up

1. Obesity is the number-one health problem in the United States today.
2. Heart attacks may be related to obesity (tobacco consumption, high blood pressure, and excessive serum triglycerides and LDL cholesterol).
3. Obesity and diabetes are caused by an excess of dietary sugars and refined starches.
4. Obesity can cause a decreased breathing ability.

5. Gallbladder disease is associated with obesity.
6. High blood pressure is aggravated by obesity.
7. Arthritic conditions could be caused or aggravated by obesity.
8. Statistics have determined that obese persons are more susceptible to having cancer.
9. The majority of obese people may be suffering from sarcopenic obesity with malnutrition and depleted muscles and other vital lean tissues.

Chapter XIII

Your Problem Of Obesity

At the end of thirteen months, Jane had lost 95 pounds. Her general emotional disposition had markedly improved and people with whom she associated had difficulty recognizing her. Her tremendous measurement of 50-43-54 had been reduced and tightened to an attractive 36-27-36. From her initial weight of 232, she had firmed down to 137. Twenty years later, she has remained a trim 135 pounds. A good number of the people I have treated have achieved this success, but all too many have not demonstrated the belief and perseverance of Jane. That is why I have written this book. I want everyone to know that there is a way.

In the preceding twelve chapters, I have done my part in bringing together the facts and in pointing out this way. Your part in solving your problem is to put this knowledge to work.

That this method can work has been demonstrated by Jane and by many others. As I write these words, I am still thrilled with the wonderful results achieved by a woman whom I saw this morning. Only ten months ago, she weighed 212 pounds, measured 44-34-44, and was a very miserable person. She told me how her husband had been very kind and understanding, but that she knew he wasn't happy with her. She was on the verge of complete despair, having spent actually thousands of dollars and endured years of misery trying to become thin. She felt unwanted and rejected, and admitted that she loathed herself. She was unable to look me in the eye and kept her glance down whenever I talked directly to her, but she got the message.

As the months went by, I could see her emerging from her cocoon of misery and today she was vivacious. She had the look of a movie star, sun-tanned in a sunsuit with purple sandals and diamond-studded light-blue sunglasses. Her personality measured 36-26-36.

It was a wonderful experience for me to realize that this woman had sought for and had entered a new world of living. Many people are not able to recognize her as the same person and have commented they thought her husband had divorced her. They recognized her poodle, but she had become another woman.

Now, let's you and I sit down together right now and take a good look at your problem and ask some questions. Have you been eating vegetable oils? Have you been eating three meals a day and two between-meal snacks a day? After breakfast have you been avoiding all fruits, sugars, refined starches, and caffeine? Have you avoided eating all carbohydrates between meals? Do you eat protein and add olive oil or canola oil on your salads at lunch and dinner? If the answer to these questions is no and the solution to your overweight problem has not been forthcoming by past methods, could it be that you have been solving your problem in the wrong way?

Let's become very fundamental. You have been told to lose weight. Everyone has been deluded into thinking that all the weight they lose is body fat. This is just not so. True, fat has weight, but not all weight is fat, and over half the weight that is lost by starvation is vital tissue—muscle, liver, kidney, blood, and so on. We surely don't want to lose that. What we actually want to lose is our excess body fat.

But how do we lose body fat? Fat can either be lost by cutting it off or by expending it as energy in the metabolic process. Surgery? No! It is much easier to increase the metabolic rate. Exercise will do this and eating certain foods will also accomplish this. In fact, it has been proven that the ingestion of certain vegetable oils, such as corn oil or olive oil in a low carbohydrate diet will increase the metabolism and loss of body fat by 20 to 25 percent. Certain drugs will likewise accomplish this goal and these may be prescribed by your doctor. And remember that fat burns fat, and the more muscle and other essential tissues you regain, the more body fat you will burn and the thinner you will get and without sagging.

Recently, a seventy-seven-year-old woman came to my office. She showed me a picture of herself when she was forty. At that time, she was a good-looking woman. I asked her how much fat she had eaten over the past thirty-seven years. She stated honestly that she had avoided eating any fat at all. She weighed 350 pounds. You be the judge.

Now, we not only want to get rid of our excess body fat, but we want to stop storing any more in our fat cells, that's for certain. Remember that every fat cell in the body is a miniature fat factory and that the manufacture of fat can take place only in the presence of insulin (secreted whenever the blood sugar rises) and alpha-glycerophosphate, a metabolite of blood sugar. Since all carbohydrates are assimilated as blood sugar, we definitely want to restrict the amount of carbohydrates in our diet.

Thus far, we have been discussing only fat. What about the real you, the inner body, muscles, liver, and other organs? Your enjoyment of life depends upon the proper function of these vital body parts.

Now, if you don't eat for several hours, your body will tear down the cells of these vital tissues and convert them into sugar to keep your brain and nervous system functioning. The body is incapable of turning your excess fat into blood sugar, the mandatory energy to your brain. This was shown in the Oakland Naval Hospital experiment mentioned in chapter 1. Sailors who starved ten days lost twenty pounds, but it was proven that thirteen pounds, or 65 percent, of the weight lost was vital body tissue. This is really astounding but true. So starvation or extreme caloric restriction is out. In fact, at this moment you may, in reality, be a thin person with a heavy fat coat, having depleted your vital tissue. This can be demonstrated by outlining the muscle of an arm with your thumbs. Many "huge" arms are found to be actually thin ones surrounded by fat.

To regain and support this vital tissue, you must have protein at each meal along with certain essential dietary fats that the body is unable to manufacture, and you must engage in active physical exercise daily.

You may have a water-retention problem. Many times this is quite complicated and demands the help of your doctor. But in general, drinking less water is not the answer. In fact, by drinking more water, you will have less tendency to hold water. Be sure to cut down on your salt intake as you regain your inner vital tissues, and the water problem may not be nearly so difficult.

By feeding the inner body then, better health, a more attractive appearance, and greater efficiency and zest for living will be yours.

Now, you must decide to put these principles into action. Your creative imagination is the tool to use. Form an image of what you want to look like in your mind's eye and keep this image there until it becomes a reality. And don't be in a hurry. It may take several months to get the job done. But it will be for good.

To do this, you should *forget about the scal*e. This has really nothing to do with how you look. A girdle will actually make you heavier by its weight. You wear a girdle because what you really want is to become slim and attractive, not lose weight. *No one knows what anyone weighs, but everyone knows what they see.* So, get out your tape measure; use it instead of a scale. When you lose inches, you will be getting the results you are actually seeking—losing body fat. Certain friends of my patients have often commented, "You look like you lost forty pounds," when the patient may have lost only twenty but several inches in every measurement.

The treatment of obesity has been very discouraging in the past because the goal of losing weight was a false one and the method of counting calories without specifying the kind of calories to be counted was very inaccurate. Look around the room you are sitting in at this moment. Everything in it has calories and weight. That hardly describes the room, though, does it?

I often relate this story to my patients. If someone came to you and said he had *a bag containing gold, sand, and sawdust* and that it weighed thirty pounds, and asked you how much you would pay for it—what would your answer be? Remember your body has three essential components: (I) vital tissue, (2) fat, and (3) water. The scale cannot differentiate among them. The way you look in the mirror and the way you feel are the best indicators of your proper weight.

Another comparison—a pound of cotton and a pound of lead weigh the same, but a pound of cotton takes up much more space. And I am sure that you have noticed that the fat globules in a bowl of soup always float on the top. Fat has a lighter density than either water or flesh, and therefore *a pound of fat takes up more space within your skin than a pound of flesh.*

On this program, you will actually be gaining on the inside—vital lean tissues—while losing the unwanted outer coat of body fat. In the beginning, the vital-tissue gain will offset the loss of fat tissue but your dimensions will be decreasing steadily from the start. As time goes on, the scale will definitely reflect the weight loss, but having regained inner vital tissue and lost body fat, you can remain trim, healthy, and attractive by staying with the method of eating outlined in Chapter 8.

On this diet, your average *weight loss will range between three to eight pounds a month.* Some will lose more, others less, but is not primarily your scale weight that is of concern. The tape measure serves a much more accurate indicator of fat loss than does the scale. Measure yourself at the chest, abdomen, and hips at least once a week. Your average loss in inches should be from one inch to three inches each month. There will be periods where you will plateau, remain at the same weight and measurements. Don't be discouraged—stay on this diet. The QQF is the way of eating that you can remain with for the rest of your life, one by which you can become trim, healthy and attractive and stay that way.

In contrast, any demonstrable weight lost by starvation methods will usually be regained, because having come to the end of a severe caloric-restriction regimen, your vital tissue will be depleted and fat will hang loosely in sagging skin. Usually, you will be pale, anemic, and appear haggard. The "demand" for better health and the rebuilding of vital-tissue structures will bring about a return to random overeating and many will find they have regained all the weight they had lost and then some. Not so at all with this method. Jane now weighs 135 pounds, has no sagging whatever, and is two pounds less than she was twenty years previously by remaining on the moderate fat and protein, low carbohydrate diet.

I will never forget a young woman who demonstrated great will power having "starved" herself for one year. When I saw her, my first thought was to recommend hospitalization. She was very pale with obvious anemia. Her facial expression was gaunt and her chest was sunken. She had lost thirty pounds but confessed that she had not reduced her hip measurements a fraction of an inch.

I sincerely desire that the message I have tried to bring forth will benefit all those who read this book. Hope and faith in the plan outlined and the development of these new eating habits will bring you the desired results. Please get this method fixed in your mind—and determine now to succeed.

I wish you success in achieving your goal of better health and appearance and all the happiness that may follow.

Postscript

The achievement of your success of becoming healthy, trim, and attractive is predicated upon three major "thought" powers: understanding, will, and imagination, and they are to be used in that order.

First, you must understand how to achieve the desired results, why this method is scientifically sound, and that it will work for YOU. The how and why have been explained. Secondly, you must exert your will in a continued and determined effort until you have become successful. If you are in normal health, you can and will succeed by applying the principles and methods given in the preceding chapters. Thirdly, you must "see" in your mind's eye what you will look like one year after you begin this program.

HE CAN WHO THINKS HE CAN. Eat the QQF way and always remember the restriction of "never after breakfast."

Please check with your family physician before beginning this or any other diet.

GEORGE EDWARD SCHAUF, M.A., M.D.
RIVERBANK, CALIFORNIA

Appendix

The Never After Breakfast Carbohydrate Counter

A. FOODS RESTRICTED TO BREAKFAST

Fresh Fruits	Household Measure	Grams of CBH
Apple	1 medium	22.0
Apricots	3 medium	14.0
Banana	1 medium	30.0
Blackberries	1 cup	19.0
Blueberries	1 cup	21.0
Boysenberries	1 cup	12.0
Cantaloupe	½ melon	14.0
Casaba melon	1 wedge	10.0
Cherries	1 cup pitted	19.7
Crabapple	1 medium	3.0
Cranberries	1 cup	11.0
Currants	1 cup	17.0
Dates	4	22.5
Figs	3 small	16.4

		Grams of CBH
Gooseberries	1 cup	12.5
Grapes Concord,	1 cup	26.7
Muscat,	1 cup	29.2
Tokay	1 cup	29.2
and Thompson seedless	1 cup	23.7
Grapefruit	½ medium	14.0
Guavas	1 medium	13.6
Honeydew Melon	1 medium wedge	11.2
Huckleberries	1 cup	20.0
Kumquats	5-6	10.0
Lemon	1 medium	6.0
Lime	1 medium	5.0
Loganberries	1 cup	22.5
Loquats	7	10.0
Mango	1 medium	24.1
Muskmelon	½ medium	8.0
Nectarine	1 medium	8.0
Orange	1 medium	16.0
Papaya	1 cup cubes	18.2
Peach	1 medium	10.0
Pears	1 medium	25.0
Persimmons	1 medium	25.0
Pineapple	1 slice	12.0
Plum	1 medium	7.0
Pomegranate	1 medium	19.7

		Grams of CBH
Raspberries	1 cup	17.0
Rhubarb	1 cup	4.0
Strawberries	1 cup	13.0
Tangerine	1 medium	10.0
Watermelon	1 medium wedge	33.2

Dried Fruits

Apples	½ cup	26.9
Apricots	3 halves	11.0
Raisins	14 cup	29.0
Peaches	½ cup	40.0
Prunes	4 medium	20.0

Canned Fruits

Applesauce, unsweetened	½ cup	10.8
Apricots, syrup pack	3 halves	22.0
Apricots, water pack	3 halves	9.8
Blackberries, syrup pack	½ cup	23.5
Blueberries, syrup pack	½ cup	30.0
Blueberries, water pack	½ cup	10.0
Cherries	½ cup	13.0
Cherries, syrup pack	1 cup	30.0
Cranberry sauce	½ cup	55.8

		Grams of CBH
Fruit cocktail in syrup	½ cup	25.0
Peaches, syrup pack	2 halves	11.6
Peaches, water pack sliced	1 cup	16.0
Pears, syrup pack	½ cup	25.0
Pears, water pack	½ cup	10.3
Pineapple, juice pack	1 large slice	21.2
Pineapple, water pack	1 large slice	10.2
Raspberries, water pack	½ cup	8.8
Plums, syrup	½ cup	26.5

Fruit Juices

Apple	¾ cup	23.9
Apricot, unsweetened	1 cup	29.2
Apricot, Nectar	¾ cup	27.0
Blackberry	1 cup	19.5
Blueberry	1 cup	34.2
Cranberry	1 cup	38.6
Grape	¾ cup	29.9
Grapefruit, unsweetened	1 cup	21.5
Lemon	1 cup	19.2
Lime	1 cup	22.5
Loganberry	1 cup	24.6

		Grams of CBH
Nectarine	1 cup	34.9
Orange	1 cup	25.8
Orange apricot	1 cup	32.0
Papaya	1 cup	30.2
Peach Nectar	1 cup	31.0
Pear Nectar	1 cup	33.0
Pineapple	1 cup	34.0
Prune	1 cup	47.5
Raspberry	1 cup	25.6
Tangerine	1 cup	25.2
Blackberries, water pack	½ cup	11.0

Jams and Jellies

Apple Butter	1 tbsp.	9.1
Blackberry Jam	1 tbsp.	14.2
Blackberry Jelly	1 tbsp.	13.0
Cranberry Jelly	1 tbsp.	10.9
Currant Jelly	1 tbsp.	13.2
Guava butter	1 tbsp.	10.0
Grape Jelly	1 tbsp.	15.0
Lemon Jelly	1 tbsp.	13.4
Orange Marmalade	1 tbsp.	14.0
Plum Jam	1 tbsp.	15.0
Preserves	1 tbsp.	14.8
Strawberry Jam	1 tbsp.	14.6

		Grams of CBH
Syrups		
Cane-sugar Syrup	1 tbsp.	12.5
Chocolate	1 tbsp.	11.7
Corn	1 tbsp.	14.8
Honey	1 tbsp.	16.4
Maple	1 tbsp.	12.8
Molasses, light	1 tbsp.	13.0
Molasses, blackstrap	1 tbsp.	11.0
sorghum	1 tbsp.	13.4
Sugars		
Beet Sugar	1 tbsp.	11.2
Brown Sugar	1 tbsp.	12.5
Confectioners'	1 tbsp.	8.0
Granulated	1 tsp. level	4.0
Granulated	1 tbsp.	11.9
Maple	1 tbsp.	10.9
Pastries		
Cream Puff	1	15.7
Danish	1 medium	22.8
Doughnut, plain	1	16.0
Doughnut, jelly	1	30.0
Doughnut, cruller	1	20.0
Eclair, Chocolate, custard	1	20.3
Eclair, chocolate, cream	1	15.7

		Grams of CBH
Pies		
Apple	1 piece	53.4
Apricot	1 piece	57.7
Banana custard	1 piece	49.2
Berry	1 piece	47.5
Blackberry	1 piece	49.0
Blueberry	1 piece	50.0
Butterscotch, whipped cream	1 piece	46.6
Cherry	1 piece	54.7
Chocolate chiffon, whipped cream	1 piece	46.2
Chocolate Meringue	1 piece	54.7
Coconut Custard	1 piece	46.2
Cream	1 piece	41.3
Custard	1 piece	35.1
Lemon Chiffon	1 piece	38.2
Lemon Meringue	1 piece	45.3
Mincemeat	1 piece	59.4
Peach	1 piece	60.0
Peach, whipped cream	1 piece	59.0
Pecan	1 piece	68.6
Pineapple	1 piece	48.2
Pineapple Cheese	1 piece	39.9
Pineapple Chiffon	1 piece	41.8
Prune	1 piece	60.9
Pumpkin	1 piece	32.4

		Grams of CBH
Raisin	1 piece	62.5
Rhubarb	1 piece	55.7
Strawberry	1 piece	54.9
Strawberry cream	1 piece	56.2

Cakes

Almond, coffee	1 piece	32.8
Angel Food	1 piece	30.1
Apple Crumb	1 piece	49.1
Applesauce	1 piece	18.7
Butter, plain	1 piece	36.3
Butter, iced	1 piece	46.1
Caramel, iced	1 piece	38.1
Cheesecake	1 piece	27.8
Chocolate, plain	1 piece	22.8
Chocolate, iced	1 piece	45.0
Chocolate layer cake	1 piece	54.8
Coconut	1 piece	50.0
Coffee, plain	1 piece	31.6
Coffee, iced with nuts	1 piece	32.8
Cupcake, plain	1	22.4
Cupcake, iced	1	31.0
Devil's food	1 piece	23.4
Foundation	1 piece	30.0
Fruit	Small piece	23.9
Gingerbread	1 square	26.9
Marble	1 slice	30.0
Nut loaf	1 piece	25.0

		Grams of CBH
Pineapple upside down	1 piece	70.0
Poundcake	1 piece	16.0
Strawberry shortcake	1 square	21.0
Sponge cake	1 small piece	23.8
Vanilla	1 piece	15.0
Washington cream	1 piece	40.0

Cookies

Animal crackers	1	1.8
Boston	1	2.5
Brownies	1	13.2
Butter	1	7.0
Butterscotch	1	14.6
Chocolate	1	5.4
Chocolate chip	1	7.4
Chocolate marshmallow	1	8.6
Coconut bar	1	7.6
Date bar	1	17.8
Devil's food square	1	11.0
Fig bar	1	9.7
Graham cracker	1	4.0
Graham cracker, chocolate covered	1	6.9
Honey	1	7.0
Ladyfinger	1 large	7.6
Lorna Doone	1	5.0

		Grams of CBH
Macaroon, coconut	1	12.1
Marshmallow	1	11.2
Molasses	1	5.0
Nabisco	1	1.8
Oatmeal	1	12.0
Oreo	1	7.0
Orange thin	1	8.0
Peanut	1	7.0
Raisin	1	12.5
Sugar wafer	1	11.0
Vanilla wafer	1	4.0
Waffle cream	1	7.2

Candies

		Grams of CBH
Bonbon	1	9.0
Brown Sugar Fudge	1 piece	22.9
Butterscotch	1 piece	4.3
Candy, hard	2 pieces	4.5
Caramel	1	7.8
Chocolate Milk	1 oz.	15.9
Chocolate Semisweet	1 oz.	17.5
Chocolate Kiss	1	2.3
Chocolate Almond	1 oz.	15.7
Chocolate Cream	1 medium	8.6
Chocolate Mints	3 small	21.6
Chocolate Fudge	1 piece	19.7
Citron candy	1 piece	22.7
Coconut	1 square	20.0

		Grams of CBH
Date Cream	½ oz. piece	10.0
Divinity Fudge	1 piece, 1 oz.	22.9
Fruit Drops	3	9.9
Glazed Fruit	1 piece, 1 oz.	8.0
Gumdrops	8 small	8.6
Jelly beans	1 0	16.7
Life Saver	1	1.0
Maple Sugar	1	23.5
Marshmallow, chocolate	1	8.6
Molasses Kiss	1	5.0
Orange Drop		3.0
Orange-peel Candy		20.0
Peanut Brittle	1 piece, 1 oz.	18.2
Peppermint Stick	1 piece, 1 oz.	17.5
Taffy, saltwater	1 kiss	6.2
Toffee, coffee	1 piece	4.5
Turkish Delight	1 square piece	4.5

Ice Cream

Banana	½ cup	18.0
Banana Split	1	94.5
Black-and-white soda	1	38.7
Butter Almond	½ cup	20.0
Butter Becan	½ cup	20.0
Caramel	½ cup	17.5
Cherry	½ cup	17.5

		Grams of CBH
Cherry Soda	1	28.3
Chocolate Chip	½ cup	22.5
Chocolate	½ cup	18.6
Chocolate soda	1	44.7
Chocolate Malt	1	55.0
Chocolate Sundae	1	50.0
Coffee	½ cup	17.4
Cone, 1 scoop	1	23.0
Dixie cup	1	16.2
Lemon ice cream	½ cup	17.5
Lemon Ice	½ cup	27.5
Orange Sherbet	½ cup	27.5
Parfait, Coffee	1	15.0
Peace Ice Cream	½ cup	17.5
Raspberry Sherbet	½ cup	27.5
Tutti-frutti	½ cup	15.0
Vanilla	½ cup	17.6
Vanilla Malt	1 10 oz.	50.0

Puddings

Apple Betty	1 cup	34.0
Apple Dumpling	1 medium	50.0
Apple Snow	½ cup	21.5
Apricot Whip	½ cup	21.2
Banana Custard	½ cup	19.2
Banana Whip	½ cup	15.5
Bavarian Orange	1 serving	39.8
Blancmange, Vanilla	½ cup	19.9
Bread with raisins	¾ cup	46.8

		Grams of CBH
Butterscotch	½ cup	28.9
Caramel	½ cup	28.9
Chocolate	½ cup	30.6
Custard	½ cup	14.0
Date torte with ice cream	½ cup	62.5
Gelatin, fruit flavors	½ cup	16.5
Junket	½ cup	8.7
Plum, no sauce	½ cup	25.0
Prune Whip	½ cup	25.0
Rice	½ cup	17.0
Tapioca	½ cup	18.0
Vanilla	½ cup	24.0

Soft Drinks

Cherry Soda	8 oz.	28.0
Coca-Cola	8 oz.	25.0
Cream Soda	8 oz.	28.0
Fruit Punch	8 oz.	42.5
Ginger Ale	8 oz.	21.0
Grape Soda	8 oz.	28.0
Lemon Soda	8 oz.	28.0
Orange Soda	8 oz.	27.0
Pepsi-Cola	8 oz.	27.6
Quinine Water	8 oz.	9.0
Root beer	8 oz.	23.7
Sarsaparilla	8 oz.	24.5

All caffeine-containing liquids, such as black coffee, strong tea, and cola-containing beverages are restricted to breakfast.

Cereals and Grains		Grams of CBH
Barely Flour	½ cup	43.0
Bran	1 cup	44.6
Bran Flakes	¾ cup	22.6
Buckwheat, flour	½ cup	39.0
Cornmeal	½ cup	45.0
Corn Flakes	1 cup	21.0
Corn Soya	¾ cup	21.0
Cracked wheat, cooked	2/3 cup	20.4
Cream of Wheat	1 cup	26.9
Hominy	¼ cup	28.4
Macaroni, cooked	1 cup	32.4
Noodles, cooked	1 cup	37.3
Oatmeal, cooked	1 cup	23.0
Oats, rolled dry	1 cup	19.0
Pancake, buckwheat	1, 4-inch diam.	10.4
Pancake, white flour	1,4-inch diam.	12.6
Rice, brown, cooked	¾ cup	32.4
Rice flakes	1 cup	27.4
Rice, white, cooked	¾ cup	33.0
Soybeans	1 cup	36.0
Spaghetti	1 cup	40.0
Wheat, all-purpose	½ cup	44.0
Waffles	1 medium	28.0
Popcorn, popped	1 cup	8.0

		Grams of CBH
Breads		
Bagel	1 medium	30.0
Biscuit	1 small	13.0
Banana bread	1 slice	22.8
Boston brown	1 slice	20.0
Bran raisin	1 slice	27.0
Brown nut	1 slice	24.0
Cinnamon bread	1 slice	16.2
Dare-nut	1 piece	28.0
Graham	1 slice	11.0
Raisin	1 slice	13.8
Rye, dark	1 slice	15.2
Rye, parry	1 oval	7.8
Vienna	1 slice	10.4
White	1 slice	11.8
Rolls		
Cloverleaf	1	20.0
Frankfurter	1	20.5
French	1	20.9
Hamburger	1	20.5
Hard	1	28.0
Parker House	1	13.5
Plain	1	20.0
Whole wheat	1	18.3

		Grams of CBH
Muffins		
Bran	1	20.0
Corn	1	18.0
English	1	17.5
Plain	1	16.0
Soy	1	16.0
Whole wheat	1	17.0

		Grams of CBH
Milk		
Buttermilk	8 oz.	12.0
Cream, Half and Half	1 cup	11.0
Evaporated	1 cup	24.0
Nonfat, dry, instant	1 cup powder	35.0
Skimmed	1 cup	12.5
Whole milk	1 cup	12.0

B. FOODS ALLOWED AT ANY MEAL

		Grams of CBH
Artichoke	1 bottom	5.0
Asparagus	6 spears	3.0
Bamboo shoots	3 ½ oz.	5.5
Bean Sprouts, soy	1 cup	5.0
Beans, Green	1 cup	7.0
Beans, lima	1 cup cooked	34.0

		Grams of CBH
Beet greens	½ cup cooked	2.5
Beets	2	7.0
Broccoli	1 stalk	6.0
Brussels Sprouts, cooked	1 cup	10.0
Cabbage, shredded	1 cup	4.0
Calabash	3 ½ oz.	2.0
Carrots, raw	1	5.0
Cauliflower, cooked	1 cup	5.0
Celery	1 large stalk	2.0
Chard, cooked	1 cup	2.0
Chives, chopped	3 ½ oz.	2.0
Chicory	5-6 leaves	2.0
Collards	1 cup	6.7
Corn	1 ear	21.4
Cucumber	1 medium	3.8
Dandelion Greens, cooked	1 cup	12.0
Eggplant, fried	1 slice	11.5
Endive	2 oz.	2.0
Garlic	1 clove	0.4
Kale, cooked	1 cup	7.0
Lettuce	1 head	8.0
Mint, chopped	1 tsp.	Trace
Mushrooms	1 cup	9.5
Mustard Greens	1 cup	6.0
Okra	9 pods	5.0
Parsley, chopped	1 tbsp.	Trace
Parsnips, cooked	½ cup	11.5

		Grams of CBH
Peas	1 cup	19.0
Pepper, green	1 medium	3.0
Pepper, red	1 medium	4.0
Potato, baked	1 medium	21.0
Potatoes, french-fried	10 pieces	20.0
Pumpkin	1 cup	18.0
Radishes	4 small	1.0
Romaine lettuce	¼ head	0.7
Rutabaga, cooked	1 cup	12.5
Sauerkraut	½ cup	4.5
Soybeans	½ cup	34.4
Snow peas	14	5.0
Spanish, cooked	1 cup	6.0
Tomato	1 medium	7.0
Squash, summer	½ cup	3.5
Squash, winter	½ cup	16.0
Sweet Potato, baked	1	28.0
Turnip Tops, cooked	½ cup	2.5
Turnips, cooked	½ cup	4.0
Watercress	1 bunch	5.0
Yams, cooked	1 cup	45.0
Zucchini, cooked	½ cup	4.0

Canned and Dry Vegetables

Asparagus, canned	6 spears	3.0
Beans, navy, dry	½ cup	61.6
Beans, pinto, dry	½ cup	63.7

		Grams of CBH
Beans, baked, canned pork and molasses	1 cup	50.0
Beans, wax, canned	1 cup	10.0
Beans, lima, canned	1 cup	34.0
Beets, canned	½ cup	9.5
Carrots, canned, diced	1 cup	10.0
Mushrooms, canned	1 cup	9.0
Peas, canned	1 cup	33.0
Pickle, sweet	1 large	2.5
Pickle, sour	1 large	3.0
Pumpkin, canned	1 cup	17.5
Soybeans, dry	½ cup	34.7
Spinach, canned	1 cup	6.0
Sweet Potatoes, canned	1 cup	54.0
Tomatoes, canned	1 cup	10.0

Crackers

Butter Thin	1	2.8
Cheese Tidbits	10	2.0
Melba Toast	1	3.9
Oyster	5	3.5
Pretzel, 3-ring	1	2.9
Ritz cheese	1	1.9
Saltine	1	2.9
Soda, unsalted	1	4.4
Whole-Wheat Thin	1	1.2
Zwieback	1	5.4

		Grams of CBH
Eggs		
Boiled	1	0.3
Creamed	2 eggs, 3 tbsp. sauce	5.1
Deviled	2 halves	0.5
Dried	1 tbsp.	0.2
Duck	1	2.4
Fried	1	2.4
Fried in vegetable oil	1	0.3
Raw	1	0.3
Raw, white	1	0.2
Raw, yolk	1	0.1
Omelet, plain-vegetable oil	1 egg	0.3
Omelet, cheese	2 eggs	0.9
Omelet, Spanish		
Cheeses		
American	1 oz.	0.6
American, grated	1 tbsp.	0.1
Blue Cheese	1 oz.	0.6
Domestic	1 oz.	0.6
Camembert	1 oz.	0.6
Chateau	1 oz.	1.0
Cheddar	1 oz.	0.6
Cheddar, grated	1 tbsp.	0.1
Cottage	½ cup	4.0

		Grams of CBH
Creamed	1 oz.	0.6
Edam	1 oz.	0.5
Farmer	1 oz.	1.0
Gorgonzola	1 oz.	0.5
Liederkranz	1 oz.	0.6
Limburger	1 oz.	0.6
Mysost	1 oz.	15.4
Neufchatel	1 oz.	2.2
Swiss	1 oz.	0.5
Yogurt	1 cup	12.7

Cheese Spreads

Bacon	1 oz.	1.9
Old English	1 oz.	1.9
Olive Pimento	1 oz.	1.9
Pimento	1 oz.	1.9
Roka, spread	1 oz.	2.0
Pineapple	1 oz.	2.9

Soups

Asparagus	¾ cup	12.9
Barley	¾ cup	18.5
Bean, navy	¾ cup	20.2
Beef Broth	¾ cup	3.7
Beef Noodle	¾ cup	4.6
Beef with Vegetable and Barley	¾ cup	6.9
Bouillon	¾ cup	0.0

		Grams of CBH
Celery, creamed	¾ cup	12.7
Chicken, creamed	¾ cup	0.0
Chicken Gumbo	¾ cup	12.2
Chicken Noodle	¾ cup	6.9
Chicken Rice	¾ cup	3.9
Chili Beef	¾ cup	18.9
Clam Chowder, with milk	¾ cup	13.5
Consommé, clear	¾ cup	0.0
Duck, creamed	¾ cup	7.5
Green Pea	¾ cup	17.9
Gumbo Creole	¾ cup	9.1
Minestrone	¾ cup	9.1
Mushroom, creamed	¾ cup	13.2
Noodle	¾ cup	6.7
Onion	¾ cup	5.2
Pea, creamed	¾ cup	20.6
Pepperpot	¾ cup	6.8
Potato, creamed	¾ cup	13.8
Rice	¾ cup	13.1
Scotch broth	¾ cup	9.0
Shrimp creamed	¾ cup	11.0
Spinach	¾ cup	10.2
Split pea	¾ cup	18.0
Tomato	¾ cup	12.1
Tomato rice	¾ cup	12.7
Turkey noodle	¾ cup	7.5
Turtle	¾ cup	7.0
Vegetable	¾ cup	10.5

		Grams of CBH
Salads		
Asparagus tips	6 spears	3.0
Avocado	½ medium, pear	6.5
Coleslaw	6 tbsp.	5.0
Chicken, with Celery	½ cup	2.5
Crab, with Celery	½ cup	3.0
Egg and Tomato	1 of each	4.1
Lettuce and Tomato	1 cup, heaped	5.4
Lobster, with Celery	½ cup	3.0
Macaroni	½ cup	24.8
Mixed Greens, with French dressing	½ cup	4.8
Salmon	½ cup	2.5
Shrimp with Celery	½ cup	1.5
Tomato with Cucumber	3 oz.	3.0
Tuna	½ cup	2.5
Vegetable, combination	½ cup	6.2
Waldorf	½ cup	9.7
Salad Dressings		
Bacon and Vinegar	1 tbsp.	0.5
Blue Cheese	1 tbsp.	1.0
French	1 tbsp.	1.0
Italian	1 tbsp.	1.0

		Grams of CBH
Mayonnaise	1 tbsp.	trace
Oils, salad or cooking	1 tbsp.	0.0
Roquefort	1 tbsp.	trace
Russian	1 tbsp.	1.0
Thousand Island	1 tbsp.	1.0
Vinegar and Oil	1 tbsp.	trace

Stews

Beef and Vegetable	1 cup	15.0
Lamb and Vegetable	1 cup	11.3
Oyster	1 cup	11.0
Rabbit	1 cup	11.3
Veal, and Vegetable	1 cup	11.3

Sauces

A-1	1 tbsp.	2.2
Barbecue	1 tbsp.	8.0
Catsup, tomato	1 tbsp.	4.0
Cheese	¼ cup	5.0
Chili	1 tbsp.	4.0
Cream sauce	1 tbsp.	1.5
Creole	¼ cup	7.8
Garlic with butter	1 tbsp.	0.5
Gravy, thick	1 tbsp.	7.5
Hollandaise	1 tbsp.	trace
Mustard	2 tbsp.	1.0
Sour cream	1 tbsp.	3.5
Soy	1 tbsp.	1.2

		Grams of CBH
Tartar	1 tbsp.	1.3
Tomato	¼ cup	5.0
White Sauce	¼ cup	3.2
Worcestershire	1 tbsp.	2.8

Meat Combinations

Chipped Beef, with Cream	½ cup	6.0
Corned Beef, and Hash	1 cup	20.0
Beef Croquette	1 medium	9.0
Liver, cooked	3 ½ oz.	6.0
Meatloaf	3 oz.	11.0
Potpie	1 5-inch diam.	40.0
Sweetbreads, creamed	½ cup	6.0
Lamb Curry	½ cup	22.0
Chicken Croquette	1 medium	7.5
Chicken a la King	½ cup	6.0
Chicken Pie	1 small	24.6
Stuffing, meat	½ cup	28.0
Turkey Pot Pie	1 5-inch diam.	44.4
Salami	4 oz.	1.5
Sausage, Polish	8 oz.	1.0
Wiener schnitzel	4 oz. slice	1.0

		Grams of CBH
Fish Combinations		
Clams, steamers, canned	4 oz.	4.0
Clams, stuff, baked	2	10.0
Codfish, creamed	1 cup	16.0
Crabmeat, canned	8 oz.	2.5
Fish Croquette	1 medium	8.0
Gefilte fish	4 oz.	10.0
Lobster Cantonese	1 serving	7.5
Oysters, stewed, creamed	1 cup	10.0
Scallops, broiled	4 oz.	2.5
Shrimp Creole	6 shrimp with sauce	18.6
Tuna casserole	1 average portion	25.0
Nuts		
Almonds	¼ cup	7.0
Brazil	6	2.4
Butternuts	4-6	1.0
Cashews	6-8	3.0
Chestnuts	5-6	13.0
Filberts	5-6	1.0
Hazelnuts	5-6	1.0
Hickory	6-7	1.0
Peanuts, shelled	¼ cup	8.2

		Grams of CBH
Peanuts, Spanish	1 tbsp.	1.2
Pecans	6 meats	0.8
Pine nuts	6-7	1.5
Pistachios	6 medium	1.6
Walnuts, black	6 meats	1.6
Walnuts, English	5-6 meats	1.4

C. ALCOHOLIC BEVERAGES

		Grams of CBH
Beers		
Ale	8 oz.	8.0
Beer	12 oz. bottle	14.0
Porter of stout	8 oz.	10.0
Cocktails, Highballs		
Alexander, gin	3 oz.	3.0
Bacardi cocktail	3 oz.	3.4
Bloody Mary	6 oz.	5.0
Bourbon and Soda	8 oz.	0.0
Bourbon and Ginger Ale	8 oz.	15.7
Cuba libre	10 oz.	10.0
Daiquiri	3 oz.	5.0
Dubonnet	3 oz.	12.0
Gin	1 ½ oz.	0.0
Gin Collins	10 oz.	6.0
Gin Fizz	10 oz.	7.0

		Grams of CBH
Gin Rickey	10 oz.	1.5
Grasshopper	3 oz.	18.0
Jack Rose	3 oz.	4.5
Manhattan	3 oz.	8.0
Martini, dry	3 oz.	0.2
Martini, sweet	3 oz.	8.0
Mint Julep	3 oz.	2.7
Old Fashioned	3 oz.	3.5
Orange Blossom	3 oz.	4.0
Pink Lady	3 oz.	3.5
Planter's Punch	3 oz.	7.9
Rum Collins	10 oz.	9.0
Rum and Cola	8 oz.	20.4
Rum Fizz	8 oz.	7.0
Rye highball, Soda	8 oz.	0.0
Rye highball, Ginger Ale	8 oz.	15.7
Scotch Manhattan	8 oz.	0.0
Scotch Mist	3 oz.	0.0
Screwdriver	8 oz.	15.0
Singapore Sling	8 oz.	15.0
Sloe Gin	1 oz.	0.0
Sloe Gin Fizz	8 oz.	1.3
Stinger	8 oz.	9.0
Tom Collins	10 oz.	9.0
Tom and Jerry	8 oz.	15.0
Whiskey fizz	8 oz.	5.0
Whiskey sour	3 oz.	4.0

		Grams of CBH
Zombi	14 oz.	25.0

Liquors, Whiskeys

Bourbon whiskey	1 ½ oz.	0.0
Canadian whiskey	1 ½ oz.	0.0
Gin	1 ½ oz.	0.0
Irish whiskey	1 ½ oz.	0.0
Rum	1 ½ oz.	0.0
Scotch	1 ½ oz.	0.0
Vodka	1 ½ oz.	0.0

Liqueurs, Brandies

Benedictine	1 oz.	6.5
Brandy, Apricot	1 oz.	0.0
Brandy, California	1 oz.	0.0
Brandy, imported	1 oz.	0.0
Chartreuse	1 oz.	6.6
Crème de Cacao	1 oz.	6.0
Crème de Menthe	1 oz.	6.0

Wines

Chablis	4 oz.	0.5
Champagne, domestic	4 oz.	3.0
Champagne, French	4 oz.	1.0
Burgundy, red	4 oz.	0.5
Claret	4 oz.	0.5
Cognac	1 oz.	0.0
Muscatel	3 ½ oz.	14.0

		Grams of CBH
Port	4 oz.	17.0
Riesling	4 oz.	2.0
Rhine	4 oz.	2.0
Sauterne	4 oz.	5.0
Vermouth, dry	4 oz.	1.2
Vermouth, sweet	3 ½ oz.	12.0

D. BETWEEN-MEAL SNACKS

		Grams of CBH
Anchovy Fillets	8	Trace
Bacon	2 strips	0.2
Caviar	1 oz.	1.1
Cheese, American cheddar, Swiss	1 oz.	0.6
Chicken	1 piece	0.0
Clam	1	0.7
Crab Salad	¼ cup	1.5
Frankfurters, Cocktail	1-2	0.4
Gefilte fish	½ oz.	1.2
Ham, boiled	1 piece	0.0
Herring, raw, pickled	1 piece	0.5
Liver, chicken	½ oz.	0.5
Lobster, cocktail	¼ cup	0.5
Meatballs, cocktail	3	0.0
Mussel, smoked	1	Trace

		Grams of CBH
Olives, green	3 large	0.3
Olives, black	3 large	0.6
Oysters, raw	1-2	2.0
Oysters, smoked	3-6	2.0
Polish Sausage	2 oz.	Trace
Pork Rinds	2-3	0.0
Salmon	¼ cup	0.0
Sardines, canned in oil	5	0.0
Shrimp	3 large	1.1
Tuna, canned	¼ cup	0.0
Vienna sausage	1 piece	trace

Meats, poultry, and fish are encouraged at each meal and need not be counted for their carbohydrate content if not listed in preceding tables.

Polyunsaturated oils—safflower oil, corn oil, soybean oil, cottonseed oil, peanut oil, and olive oil—are to be taken at the noon and evening meals and have no carbohydrate content.

Professional Presentation of The QQF Theory Of Obesity

Major Presentations

120th Annual Convention of the American Medical Association

121st Annual Convention of the American Medical Association

26th Annual Scientific Assembly of the American Academy of Family Physicians

23rd Annual Scientific Meeting of the American Society of Clinical Hypnosis

47th Anniversary Congress of the Pan American Medical Association

50th Anniversary Congress of the Pan American Medical Association

Annual Meeting of the American Society of Bariatric Physicians

Annual Meeting of the American Geriatrics Society

Annual Meeting of the Indiana Dietetic Association

Annual Meeting of the Arizona Dietetic Association

Annual Congress of Abdominal Surgeons

Major Media Presentation
Audio Digest, California Medical Association
House Calls (call-in radio program)

Major Periodical Publications (By And About)
American Journal of Clinical Nutrition
A.M.A. News
AP Wire Services
Catholic Digest
Family Practice News
Gannett News Services
Internal Medicine News
Journal of the International Academy of Preventative Medicine
Journal of the American Geriatrics Society
Medical Tribune
Nutrition Today
Obesity and Bariatric Medicine
OB/GYN News
Science Digest
The ACA Journal of Chiropractic
UPI Wire Service
U.S. Medicine News

Dr. George Edward Schauf MA, MD, has practiced medicine for over fifty years and is the author of the books Think, Eat and Lose Fat (Information, Inc., 1970) and Think Thin (Fawcett, 1976).

Dr. Schauf began formulating the QQF Theory for the etiology of obesity in the late 1960s. Among its first champions was Jack LaLanne, for whom Dr. Schauf wrote the nutritional component of the "Power of Thinking Thin Program." He appeared on television with LaLanne, and the dietary material was distributed in booklet and audio form.

Dr. Schauf first presented his QQF Theory of Obesity, challenging the validity of the traditionally accepted Caloric Theory, at the 120th and 121st Annual Conventions of the American Medical Association. The QQF Theory was then presented at several national medical meetings including the 26th Annual Scientific Assembly of the American Academy of Family Physicians and 50th Anniversary Congress of the Pan American Medical Association. It was reported in a variety of national news media including UPI and AP Wire Services, Consumer's Guide, Gannett News Services, A.M.A. News, US Medicine News, Internal Medicine News, and Family Practice News.

The QQF Theory was first published in the Journal of the American Geriatrics Society in 1973. It was then published in the Journal of the International Academy of Preventative Medicine in 1976. In 2006, it was published in the American Journal of Bariatric Medicine, the Bariatrician. Drawing the interest of practitioners worldwide, Dr. Schauf extensively presented his theory into the 1980s. All the while, he continued in his family practice and his successful treatment of obese patients.

After studying Engineering for three years at Santa Clara University, Dr. Schauf earned his BA and MA in Psychology from San Jose State University. He earned his MD from St. Louis University School of Medicine in 1957. A Diplomat of the American Board of Family Practice, the American Board of Bariatric Medicine, the National Board of Medical Examiners, he is a Charter Fellow and Lifetime

Member of the American Academy of Family Physicians and past member of the American Society of Clinical Hypnosis. He is a member of the California Medical Association and the American Medical Association. In 1996, the American Board of Family Practice honored Dr. Schauf with its Award of Merit.

Dr. George E. Schauf, M.D., retired after fifty-three years in Medical practice, and forty-five years in Bariatric medicine from Riverbank, CA.